MORE 4U!

theclinics.com

This Clinics series is available online.

Here's what you get:

- Full text of EVERY issue from 2002 to NOW
- Figures, tables, drawings, references and more
- Searchable: find what you need fast

  Search | All Clinics ▼ | for [   ] | GO |

- Linked to MEDLINE and Elsevier journals
- E-alerts

INDIVIDUAL SUBSCRIBERS

LOG ON TODAY. IT'S FAST AND EASY.

Click **Register** and follow instructions

You'll need your account number

Your subscriber account number is on your mailing label

This is your copy of:

THE CLINICS OF NORTH AMERICA

CXXX **2296532-2** 2 Mar 05

J.H. DOE, MD
531 MAIN STREET
CENTER CITY, NY 10001-001

BOUGHT A SINGLE ISSUE? Sorry, you won't be able to access full text online. Pl~~~~~~ today to get complete cont~~~~ ~~~~ervice at 800 645 2452~~~~ ~~~~4000 (outside US and Canada~~~~ ~~~~ier.com.

NEW!

Now also ~~~~~~~~ for INSTITUTIONS

Works/Integrates with MD Consult
Available in a variety of packages: Collections containing 14, 31 or 50 Clinics titles
Or Collection upgrade for existing MD Consult customers

ELSEVIER

Call today! 877-857-1047 or e-mail: mdc.groupinfo@elsevier.com

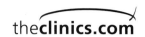

CLINICS IN PODIATRIC MEDICINE AND SURGERY OF NORTH AMERICA

Pedal Amputations

GUEST EDITOR
George F. Wallace, DPM, MBA

CONSULTING EDITOR
Vincent J. Mandracchia, DPM, MS

July 2005 • Volume 22 • Number 3

SAUNDERS

An Imprint of Elsevier, Inc.
PHILADELPHIA   LONDON   TORONTO   MONTREAL   SYDNEY   TOKYO

W.B. SAUNDERS COMPANY
A Division of Elsevier Inc.

1600 John F. Kennedy Blvd., Suite 1800, Philadelphia, PA 19103-2899

http://www.theclinics.com

**CLINICS IN PODIATRIC MEDICINE
AND SURGERY**   Volume 22, Number 3
July 2005   ISSN 0891-8422
Editor: Karen Sorensen   ISBN 1-4160-2708-4

Reprints. For copies of 100 or more of articles in this publication, please contact the Commercial Reprints Department, Elsevier Inc., 360 Park Avenue South, New York, New York 10010-1710 Tel.: (212) 633-3813, Fax: (212) 462-1935, e-mail: reprints@elsevier.com

Clinics in Podiatric Medicine and Surgery (ISSN 0891-8422) is published quarterly by Elsevier. Corporate and editorial Offices: 1600 John F. Kennedy Blvd., Suite 1800, Philadelphia, PA 19103-2899. Accounting and circulation offices: 6277 Sea Harbor Drive, Orlando, FL 32887–4800. Periodicals postage paid at Orlando, FL 32862, and additional mailing offices. Subscription prices are $170.00 per year for US individuals, $266.00 per year for US institutions, $85.00 per year for US students and residents, $205.00 per year for Canadian individuals, $322.00 per year for Canadian institutions, $225.00 for international individuals, $322.00 for international institutions and $113.00 per year for Canadian and foreign students/residents. To receive student/resident rate, orders must be accompanied by name of affiliated institution, date of term, and the *signature* of program/residency coordinator on institution letterhead. Orders will be billed at individual rate until proof of status is received. Foreign air speed delivery is included in all *Clinics* subscription prices. All prices are subject to change without notice. POSTMASTER: Send address changes to *Clinics in Podiatric Medicine and Surgery*, W.B. Saunders Company, Periodicals Fulfillment, Orlando, FL 32887-4800. **Customer Service: 1-800-654-2452 (US). From outside of the US, call 1-407-345-1000.**

Clinics in Podiatric Medicine and Surgery is covered in *Index Medicus* and *EMBASE/Excerpta Medica.*

Printed in the United States of America.

CONSULTING EDITOR

VINCENT J. MANDRACCHIA, DPM, MS, Section Chief, Podiatric Surgery, Department of Surgery, Broadlawns Medical Center; and Clinical Professor, Department of Podiatric Medicine and Surgery, College of Podiatric Medicine and Surgery, Des Moines University–Osteopathic Medicine Center, Des Moines, Iowa

GUEST EDITOR

GEORGE F. WALLACE, DPM, MBA, Director, Podiatry Service, University Hospital–University of Medicine and Dentistry of New Jersey, Newark, New Jersey

CONTRIBUTORS

GREG D. CLARK, DPM, Third Year Podiatry Resident, University Hospital–University of Medicine and Dentistry of New Jersey, Newark, New Jersey

KEITH D. COOK, DPM, Assistant Director, Podiatry Service, University Hospital–University of Medicine and Dentistry of New Jersey, Newark, New Jersey

MARK A. DeCOTIIS, DPM, Podiatry Service, University Hospital–University of Medicine and Dentistry of New Jersey, Newark; and Curative Wound Care Center, Bayshore Hospital, Holmdel, New Jersey

BRAJESH K. LAL, MD, Assistant Professor of Surgery, Division of Vascular Surgery, New Jersey Medical School, University Hospital–University of Medicine and Dentistry of New Jersey, Newark, New Jersey

ERIC LUI, DPM, Third Year Podiatry Resident, University Hospital–University of Medicine and Dentistry of New Jersey, Newark, New Jersey

AMANDA MESZAROS, DPM, Second Year Resident, Section of Podiatry, Department of Surgery, St. Vincent Charity Hospital, Cleveland, Ohio

CASEY J. O'DONNELL, DO, Resident Physician, Department of Physical Medicine and Rehabilitation, New Jersey Medical School, University Hospital–University of Medicine and Dentistry of New Jersey, Newark, New Jersey

FRANK T. PADBERG, Jr, MD, Professor of Surgery, Division of Vascular Surgery, New Jersey Medical School, University Hospital–University of Medicine and Dentistry of New Jersey, Newark, New Jersey; Chief, Section of Vascular Surgery, Veterans Affairs New Jersey Health Care Systems, East Orange, New Jersey

PETER J. PAPPAS, MD, Professor of Surgery and Chief, Division of Vascular Surgery, New Jersey Medical School, University Hospital–University of Medicine and Dentistry of New Jersey, Newark, New Jersey

RITCHARD C. ROSEN, DPM, FACFAS, FAPWCA, Chief, Podiatric Surgery, Holy Name Hospital, Teaneck, New Jersey; Clinical Faculty, University Hospital–University of Medicine and Dentistry of New Jersey, Newark, New Jersey; Diplomate, American Board of Podiatric Surgery, San Francisco, California

THERESA L. SCHINKE, DPM, Third Year Resident, Section of Podiatry, Department of Surgery, St. Vincent Charity Hospital, Cleveland, Ohio

JOHN J. STAPLETON, DPM, Second-Year Foot and Ankle Surgical Resident, Podiatry Service, University Hospital–University of Medicine and Dentistry of New Jersey, Newark, New Jersey

JAMES P. SULLIVAN, DPM, FACFAS, DABPS, Section Chairman, Podiatric Medicine and Surgery, Department of Orthopaedics, Jersey Shore University Medical Center, Neptune, New Jersey

GEORGE F. WALLACE, DPM, MBA, Director, Podiatry Service, University Hospital–University of Medicine and Dentistry of New Jersey, Newark, New Jersey

PETER P. YONCLAS, MD, Assistant Professor, Department of Physical Medicine and Rehabilitation, New Jersey Medical School, University Hospital–University of Medicine and Dentistry of New Jersey, Newark, New Jersey

GERARD V. YU, DPM, FACFAS, Podiatric Surgery Residency Program Chief, Section of Podiatry, Department of Surgery, St. Vincent Charity Hospital, Cleveland, Ohio; and Permanent Faculty Member and Director of Program Development, The Podiatry Institute, Tucker, Georgia

ROBERT W. ZICKLER, MD, Assistant Professor of Surgery, Division of Vascular Surgery, New Jersey Medical School, University Hospital–University of Medicine and Dentistry of New Jersey, Newark, New Jersey

CONTENTS

Amputation may take a psychological toll on a patient. Proper documentation is paramount along with a lucid informed consent. Various pathologies may lead to an amputation. Tools to aid in the decision to amputate, in choosing the levels of amputation, and in the selection of the type of procedure are available. The key to any amputation is to be at a level that is most definitive.

When performing a pedal amputation, proper preoperative, intraoperative, and postoperative care is essential for a successful outcome. This article outlines proper perioperative management for the amputation patient. All patients require appropriate medical management and testing before any surgical procedure; however, preoperative planning specific for the amputation patient also is required to determine the appropriate level of amputation and to provide an optimal result. The surgeon always must remember that patients with more distal amputations have a decreased energy expenditure and better functional outcome compared with their more proximal counterparts. Appropriate psychological counseling and physical rehabilitation also should be initiated as early as possible for the patient to recover fully in a timely fashion.

partial foot amputation offers the potential for retention of plantar load-bearing tissues that are capable of tolerating the forces involved in weight bearing; this can allow the patient to ambulate with or without a prosthesis. Because of the complexity of the foot-ankle complex and the multiple types of partial foot amputations encountered, choosing the appropriate prosthesis can be challenging. This article explains some of the rationale and common options available for the different levels of amputation.

FORTHCOMING ISSUES

January 2006
Diagnosis and Treatment of Peripheral Nerve Entrapments and Neuropathy
Babak Baravarian, DPM, *Guest Editor*

April 2006
Pediatric Foot and Ankle Disorders
Jonathan Labovitz, DPM, FACFAS, *Guest Editor*

July 2006
Implants in Foot and Ankle Surgery: Pros and Cons
Jesse B. Burks, DPM, MS, FACFAS, *Guest Editor*

RECENT ISSUES

April 2005
Osteotomies of the Foot and Ankle
D. Martin Chaney, DPM, FACFAS, *Guest Editor*

January 2005
Heel Pain
Thomas Zgonis, DPM, and
Gary Peter Jolly, DPM, *Guest Editors*

October 2004
McCarthy's Principles and Practice of Podiatric Onychopathy
Myron A. Bodman, DPM, and
Daniel J. McCarthy, DPM, PhD, *Guest Editors*

THE CLINICS ARE NOW AVAILABLE ONLINE!

http://www.theclinics.com

ELSEVIER
SAUNDERS

Clin Podiatr Med Surg
22 (2005) xi–xii

CLINICS IN
PODIATRIC
MEDICINE AND
SURGERY

Foreword

Pedal Amputations

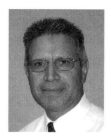

Vincent J. Mandracchia, DPM, MS
Consulting Editor

Read, read, read. Read everything—trash, classics, good and bad, and see how they do it. Just like a carpenter who works as an apprentice and studies the master. Read! You'll absorb it. Then write. If it is good, you'll find out. If it's not, throw it out the window.

—William Faulkner

Be a sponge, absorb everything, and then squeeze out what you don't want.

—Denise M. Mandi, DPM

I am impressed with the designation in our profession of the "master surgeon" and continuing medical education–sanctioned courses of the same title. The definition of a *master* is one who is skilled and proficient and is often used in combination as a descriptive term. At some point in our professional lives, I firmly believe in that moniker, especially with the accumulation of years of experience and the continuation of lifelong learning skills.

But what of the terms *apprentice* and *journeyman*? *Webster's* dictionary defines an apprentice as "an inexperienced person; one bound to another for a prescribed period with a view to learning an art or trade; one who is learning by practical experience under skilled workers a trade, art, or calling." A journeyman is defined

doi:10.1016/j.cpm.2005.03.009
podiatric.theclinics.com

as "an experienced, reliable worker." Aren't these the descriptions of what residency training is all about? I think it's time to revisit the terms *apprentice, journeyman*, and *master* and apply them to our professional preparation and achievement. We certainly have no problem referring to ourselves as master surgeons, and rightly so—but we would recoil from calling our training process an apprenticeship. However, I believe that a return to that title would help our graduating students better understand what to expect and conversely what is expected of them.

How many of us have had a mentor during our training? We try to be like them in many ways. We learn so much from them both professionally and personally. We spend as much time with them as possible and quite literally apprentice with them. As Gilbert Chesterton stated, "Education is simply the soul of a society as it passes from one generation to another." Recognizing an apprentice status could severely restrict the ego trip that some residents experience. After all, being an apprentice doesn't sound as impressive as being a resident. Just imagine what would happen to all of those "doctor" television programs. Certainly some attending might envision a Donald Trump moment with "You're fired!" being directed to the resident. But the premise is sound. Being an apprentice sets the stage for an absorptive learning process, a desire to achieve the "master" status of one's mentor.

The completion of apprentice training would allow a surgeon the title of journeyman or a reliable experienced practitioner. Announcing one's self as a journeyman surgeon would better answer the question "How long have you been practicing?" It's a better descriptor of preparative training. Certainly, a journeyman electrician is more qualified than an apprentice electrician. And with the completion of apprentice training, one truly is beginning a professional journey toward the goal of becoming a master.

By recognizing the apprentice and journeyman status of their professional training, surgeons will be humbled when they finally achieve the title of master. Its not surprising that master and mentor start with "m" and have the same number of letters. Before we can achieve the title of master, we must earn it. More importantly, we must accept the title with all of its responsibilities—are we willing to be the mentor, to teach the apprentices, to pass on the skills and experience we have achieved? Without that educational commitment, we can never really call ourselves master surgeons.

It's time for our profession to set the standard in residency training. We have already adopted the title *master surgeon*—now it is time to drop the word *residency* and return to the more descriptive terms of *apprentice* and *journeyman* practitioner. Let's "step up to the plate" and allow our graduating students the opportunity to learn their trade in an environment that promotes learning as a whole, to become like the mentor, and to be a true master.

Vincent J. Mandracchia, DPM, MS
Broadlawns Medical Center
1801 Hickman Road
Des Moines, IA 50314, USA
E-mail address: vmandracchia@broadlawns.org

ELSEVIER
SAUNDERS

Clin Podiatr Med Surg
22 (2005) xiii

CLINICS IN
PODIATRIC
MEDICINE AND
SURGERY

Preface

Pedal Amputations

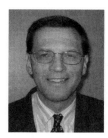

George F. Wallace, DPM, MBA
Guest Editor

With the pandemic of diabetes mellitus just beginning, podiatric physicians will see more patients with diabetic foot pathology. Some patients will require a pedal amputation. Additionally, podiatric physicians may be consulted for trauma cases that are nonsalvageable and lead to an amputation.

This issue provides some valuable insights into the perioperative and intra-operative realm of the pedal amputation patient. University Hospital–UMDNJ provides the setting and authors for the cases contained in the discussions. Be-cause of licensing constraints, the Syme's ankle disarticulation article is by Dr. Yu and involves cases from his institution.

Any attempt to compile an undertaking of this magnitude takes dedication, time, and perseverance. Everyone involved did just that and more. My gratitude is theirs for a job well done. I hope you will find this issue an informative and valuable reference.

George F. Wallace, DPM, MBA
Podiatry Service
University Hospital–University of Medicine and
Dentistry of New Jersey
150 Bergen Street, A-226
Newark, NJ 07103, USA
E-mail address: WALLACGF@UMDNJ.edu

0891-8422/05/$ – see front matter © 2005 Elsevier Inc. All rights reserved.
doi:10.1016/j.cpm.2005.03.010
podiatric.theclinics.com

ELSEVIER
SAUNDERS

Clin Podiatr Med Surg
22 (2005) 315–328

CLINICS IN
PODIATRIC
MEDICINE AND
SURGERY

Indications for Amputations

George F. Wallace, DPM, MBA

*Podiatry Service, University Hospital–University of Medicine and Dentistry of New Jersey,
150 Bergen Street, A-226, Newark, NJ 07103, USA*

The term *amputation* is defined as "the cutting off of a limb or part of a limb" [1]. A podiatric physician may be called in to evaluate a severely traumatized foot that is not salvageable. A diabetic patient presents with a grossly infected forefoot, which necessitates an open transmetatarsal amputation (TMA). Both of these scenarios are clearly described, and the need for amputation is a given. What other types of cases may result in the podiatric physician considering an amputation? Are there any diagnostic modalities or parameters available that can be used in deciding not only whether an amputation is indicated, but also at what level?

Healthy People 2000 had as one of its goals the reduction of pedal amputations secondary to diabetes. With the advent of the diabetic pandemic, the target reduction of 4.9/1000 was not met [2]. Diabetes is the leading cause of non-traumatic amputations performed in the United States [3].

Amputations can be a partial toe, a digital disarticulation, a ray or rays, a TMA, midfoot disarticulations, or a Symes (Box 1). Symes amputation is a complete amputation of the foot via disarticulation at the ankle. A guillotine amputation implies a dorsal-to-plantar amputation at any level without any flap remaining for closure. When ready to close, either a skin graft or further resection to a level where flaps are created becomes necessary.

A primary amputation is one that is completed at initial presentation. An example is a severe crush injury without any ability to save the part. The level of amputation depends on the pathology, extent of damage, functional capacity, and making a concerted effort not to "whittle" the foot by numerous surgeries. "Whittling" the foot removes a little more of the foot each time, which could continue until one determines that the only viable procedure would be either a below-knee amputation or above-knee amputation. Although there are circum-

---

E-mail address: WALLACGF@UMDNJ.edu

Box 1. Levels of amputations

Terminal Symes
Toe (partial/complete/multiples)
Ray (partial/complete/multiples)
Transmetatarsal
Lisfranc's
Chopart's
Symes's, Boyd, Pirgoff
Below-knee (transtibial)
Above-knee (transfemur)

Note: Disarticulations can occur through most joint(s). Guillotine amputations are performed at any level.

---

stances where multiple amputations are performed, it would be more prudent, with the best interest of the patient in mind, to do one definitive amputation.

Psychology and amputations

No patient wants to lose a foot no matter if the extent of damage leads to no other alternative than an amputation. Numerous psychological issues can be encountered as the procedure is explained, as it is performed, and during convalescence [4]. The psychological status of the patient has to be monitored as closely as the laboratory values.

In addition to the medical consequences of the surgery, the following psychological aspects need to be considered after determining a patient requires an amputation: Presurgical counseling with a religious cleric or bereavement counselor, social services evaluation, psychiatric evaluation, candid discussions with the patient, and clearly written consents. Preplanning on the part of the physician helps in preparing the patient, not only for the surgery, but also for life after the surgery (Fig. 1). With some patients, it may be appropriate to suggest a visit by a member of the clergy or a bereavement counselor. Input from such an individual may hasten a return to mental health and possibly prevent depression. With Health Insurance Portability and Accountability Act regulations now in place, the information that is relayed to a friend or family member has to be scrutinized.

Occasionally a patient may refuse an amputation or leave the hospital prematurely. Both situations require charting that such an action is against medical advice. In cases in which a patient may seem not to be competent to make decisions, a psychiatric consultation may be warranted. Sometimes a judge may have to become involved to declare a patient incompetent so that the proper

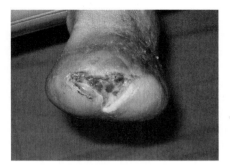

Fig. 1. Residual diabetic foot infection post TMA. Consents always should include the possibility of an amputation.

procedure can be performed. The proper protocol for such an action is contained in the administrative policies of each hospital.

Some patients, diabetics especially, have heard stories of how an amputated toe led to a few more surgeries, then the foot, the leg, and subsequently death. The fear of multiple surgeries is real with these patients when they are told an amputation will be performed. It becomes incumbent on the physician to choose the amputation site that has the greatest probability to heal. As a result of unforeseen circumstances, occasions arise when a more proximal level has to be amputated. Candid explanations and effective communication with the patient go a long way in seeing the patient through these difficult times.

Social services may have to be contacted for an evaluation. This service determines if a need exists for a home health aide or for a rehabilitation facility after discharge.

Proper documentation is paramount to lessening legal ramifications of any patient contact. This is especially true when an amputation may be a possibility or will definitely occur. One needs to document the findings, the proposed treatment, why it was selected, the explanation given to the patient, the patient's response and concerns, and any adverse effects. Additionally the current demeanor of the patient should be documented. Amputation is not an afterthought, and it should not be taken lightly by the physician or the patient. All of this should be reflected in the chart.

Consents for surgery are in lay terms [5]. Various institutions require certain verbiage and parameters to be on every consent form. At the author's institution, not only is the procedure listed, but also the risks and benefits, along with a notation of any risks of not having the proposed procedures. Alternative treatments and their specific risks and benefits are listed. Some instances may have "none" as the entry. An example is a toe with wet gangrene, which cannot be treated with conservative care.

Consents for a diabetic who presents with an infection can be problematic. The extent of the infection may not be so readily apparent despite a thorough workup (Fig. 1). It is suggested that when performing an incision and drainage on a diabetic especially, the words "amputation of toe(s) or other parts of the foot as necessary" always should appear. Such verbiage may ameliorate invoking the clause on the consent where any procedure could be performed if unforeseen circumstances occur intraoperatively. A trauma patient with a severe crush injury should have the same words in the procedure section.

Explaining the possibility of an amputation or definitely stating one will be performed has to be without equivocation and simply stated. The physician has to be ready for the possibility of numerous questions and possibly tears. These reactions must never alter the treatment.

Should the patient request a second opinion, it must be granted. It may be helpful to bring in another physician who would corroborate the need for the amputation. These steps must be performed rapidly and without hesitation when time is of the essence.

Clinical entities for amputations

The podiatric physician can be faced with myriad clinical circumstances that would necessitate an amputation (Box 2). Basically the list can be divided in two: diabetic and nondiabetic entities.

A diabetic patient can present in many ways: (1) an infection with or without an ulcer, (2) a retained foreign body, (3) in association with peripheral vascular disease initially seen with either wet or dry gangrene, (4) Charcot neuroarthropathy, (5) acute osteomyelitis or chronic osteomyelitis, and (6) after open reduction internal fixation of an ankle fracture with a postoperative infection [6]. A patient with diabetes also may present with peripheral neuropathy, which, along with the depressed immune response, may hamper healing. Naturally the podiatric physician has to decide the proper level of amputation. The initial amputation level may not be the ultimate one; this would be predicated on how well the amputation eradicates the infection, the viability of the tissue to permit

---

Box 2. General diagnoses for amputations

Diabetic foot infection
Charcot neuroarthropathy
Gangrene/peripheral vascular disease
Frostbite
Congenital
Trauma
Tumors
Osteomyelitis
Failed surgery
Intractable pain

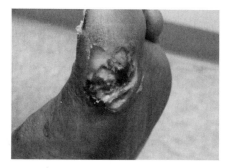

Fig. 2. Plantar ulcer, which has to be monitored closely.

healing, and functionality. After the original examination, four toes may have to be disarticulated. After hospitalization and wound care, however, the remaining toe also should be removed most likely with a standard TMA.

An ulcer that has been stable and appears to be healing suddenly can turn into a raging infection (Fig. 2). A part of the foot then is amputated because of the presence of necrotic tissue, purulence, dysvascularity, and even soft, nonviable bone. Wet gangrene also can develop with ulceration resulting in subsequent amputation. Central plantar space infections tracking along the long flexors and up into the distal part of the lower leg can be an early indication for a more proximal amputation.

Insensate diabetics may step on a foreign body that may or may not be evident on radiographic examination. An infection ensues, and a part is unsalvageable. There may not be a quantifiable immune response (Fig. 3) [7].

One or more toes may appear dusky or develop dry gangrene. Pedal pulses are absent, and arterial studies depict a peripheral blockage. Vascular surgeons are able either to bypass the stenosis or to perform an endarterectomy. The overall vascular status of the foot improves, but the gangrenous part will never reverse (Fig. 4). The best time to perform this amputation according to a study by Arroyo et al [8] would be 72 hours after the vascular surgery when the vessels show continuous patency.

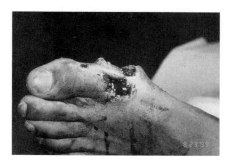

Fig. 3. Foreign body (gunshot wound) in a diabetic can be problematic.

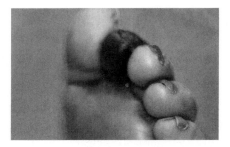

Fig. 4. Gangrene after bypass.

If there is minimal or no bleeding intraoperatively when performing either an incision and drainage or an amputation, a vascular surgery consultation is warranted. When encountering poor bleeding, the realization must be entertained that the current surgery and level of amputation may fail.

Strides in the surgical management of Charcot neuroarthropathy have given patients another option to stabilize their foot [9]. The price to pay for failures may be an amputation. Patients have to be well aware of this possiblilty before agreeing to this type of surgery (Fig. 5) [10].

Frostbite also may lead to amputations. The adage "January's frostbite is July's amputation" is prophetic. A patient with a cold injury may be seen initially with only one or two toes affected. The extent of the cold exposure and tissue damage may progress. If one is too hasty to amputate, there may be additional amputations as more tissue dies. In the absence of wet gangrene, which requires immediate amputation, the frostbitten part should be allowed to demarcate. Practically, demarcation comes before July or even before an autoamputation (Fig. 6). At the demarcated end point, an amputation can be performed or the toe will autoamputate. The latter can be a slow process, can become infected at any time, and is unsightly to the patient. Amputation via surgery eliminates the aforementioned sequence.

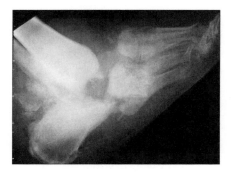

Fig. 5. Charcot's neuroarthropathy. Reconstruction failures may lead to an amputation.

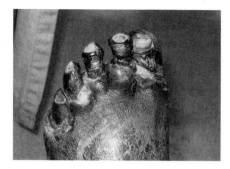

Fig. 6. Frostbite with dry and wet gangrene requiring a TMA.

Congenital pedal malformations may have no other option but amputation. A child with polydactyly either wears accommodative shoes or the extra toe is ablated. The most medial or lateral toe is not the one removed in all cases; rather, the decision is based on function and underlying osseous tissue [11]. There is no consensus as to what age the surgery is performed. When osseous structures are developed and closer to skeletal maturity, the surgery is easier (Fig. 7).

Pedal trauma can lead to an amputated part either initially or for postinjury complications. The former occurs most likely after a crush injury to the toes or foot. One or more are blatantly not viable. Pallor, Gustilo open fracture classification of IIIB and IIIC, and a toe attached literally by a thread of an anatomic part all can lead to emergent amputation [12]. Any part of the foot can be similarly affected (Fig. 8).

Complications after the injury and any trauma surgery also can lead to an amputation. As a result of the inability to decide whether to amputate, the part, which once was thought to be viable, has lost blood supply. Internal fixation failure, osteomyelitis, unremitting pain, and an insensate foot can occur anytime after pedal trauma [13]. A grossly contaminated open fracture may become so infected that no course of therapy short of amputation would be beneficial

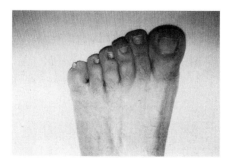

Fig. 7. Polydactyly.

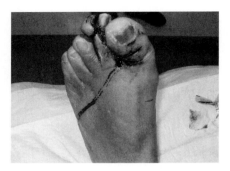

Fig. 8. Trauma leading to an amputation. Gunshot wound rendered distal aspect of second toe nonsalvageable.

to the health of the patient. Amputation may be the quickest, easiest, and least costly alternative.

Benign and malignant tumors, depending on their histologic classification and location, sometimes do not allow excision, but require an amputation, especially benign tumors encompassing an entire toe or malignant tumors in which amputation is the best treatment for long-term survival. Skin malignancies (eg, a subungual melanoma) may lead to amputation via a metatarsophalangeal disarticulation (Fig. 9) [14].

Acute osteomyelitis of the foot usually is from direct extension, whether from an overlying ulcer or from any surgery. Decompression and saucerization of the infected bone, when possible, followed by many weeks of intravenous antibiotics are the standards of treatment [15]. When confronted with an isolated toe with osteomyelitis, the surgical part to be removed may create an unviable toe. It may be better to amputate the entire toe. Chronic osteomyelitis likewise may lead to the same outcome. In situations in which excision of infected bone can be performed, it is preferable that the rest of the foot be saved (Fig. 10).

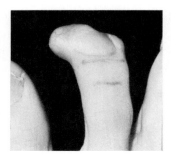

Fig. 9. Tumor (osteochondroma) leading to a distal Symes amputation.

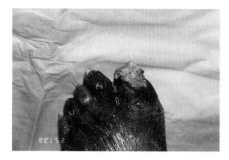

Fig. 10. Chronic osteomyelitis of hallux, which necessitated an amputation.

Any surgery can go radically wrong. A part not being viable, failure of fixation, a postoperative infection, and osteomyelitis are some instances in which amputation results. Examples are a brachymetatarsia surgery that overlengthens the shortened toe and causes vascular compromise and any postoperative infection so severe that the part has to be eliminated. These situations are relatively rare, but patients need to be forewarned via the consent process if, with a surgical procedure, such a risk exists. Another indication for an amputation, especially proximally, would be intractable pain for which all conservative measures have failed. The pain is neurogenic in origin [16].

Emergency amputations

A diabetic patient with gas in the tissues, general malaise, a temperature, and an elevated white blood cell count is a candidate for an immediate incision and drainage. Because of immunodeficiencies, however, gas may be the only finding. The areas affected may be beyond salvage. The decision to amputate is made quickly. These patients may need amputations that are not at a conventional level. The emergency amputation may be a guillotine and more proximal than previously thought. The surgeon has to decompress the area. Functional considerations are not paramount at this point. At the time of closure or skin graft, the original site can be converted to a more conventional amputation. Functional considerations are considered at this time, and appropriate procedures performed (ie, tendon balance). Any bone exposed within any wound has to be resected to healthy bone before any closure.

A patient with a crush injury presents with nonviable tissue and an open fracture. The open fracture constitutes an emergency. The presence of a part of the foot deemed not salvageable would require an emergency amputation.

Dry gangrene, which implies demarcation at least for the time, is not a reason to perform an emergency surgery. One can wait for autoamputation or perform the amputation on an elective basis. If the dry gangrenous part turns into wet gangrene, the amputation proceeds without hesitation.

Diagnostic aids to determine when an amputation is indicated

No one diagnostic aid unequivocally points to an amputation. The presence of dry or wet gangrene or dysvascularity can lead to an amputation. The surgeon's experience may dictate what can or cannot heal. The two most salient questions posed are: (1) Could the part or area in question survive as is? (2) Would the patient be better served to have the part removed? Some preoperative planning, when one looks at the diseased part, has to occur, and the patient needs to be informed [17].

Radiographs depicting the presence of a tumor or osteomyelitis may help determine preoperatively the need for an amputation. Bone scans and MRI as adjunctive tests also can be used.

The ankle-brachial index can provide a numerical measure of the ability to heal at a specific site. Values less than 0.45 have proved to be a reliable predictor of nonhealing [18]. Any reading less than 1 is a cause for alarm. Transcutaneous oxygen levels also are used and can be obtained adjacent to a nonhealing wound. Readings less than 40 mm Hg are a poor predictor of healing [19]. After any vascular intervention, numerical readings of both of these tests should improve. Failure to reach values conducive to healing would result in an amputation. Levels of amputation can be determined using these simple noninvasive vascular studies (Fig. 11).

Diabetics do not always have a leukocytosis or elevated temperature in the presence of an infection [20]. What can appear to be on the surface and systemically a "minor" infection is just the opposite when the initial incision is made. The surgeon is faced with copious purulence, necrotic tissue, and parts of a foot that are encompassed by the infection. Antibiotics alone would never eradicate this type of presentation. All nonvisible tissue, including bone, is excised. Aggressive débridement can result in a toe that intraoperatively becomes dusky, cool, flail, and nonviable. As previously discussed, when dealing with a seemingly nondescript diabetic infection, "amputation" is included in the consent.

Besides clinical assessment, a few other diagnostic schemes can be employed for trauma to the foot and lower extremity. Radiographs, CT scans, and hand-held

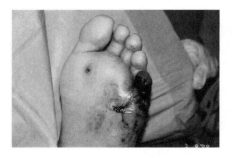

Fig. 11. Pulse volume recordings and ankle-brachial indices diminished. Distal bypass was performed.

Dopplers are a few invaluable noninvasive tools. An arteriogram should be ordered if one suspects vascular injury. With an insensate plantar surface, consideration for immediate amputation is not outside of treatment possibilities.

Two scoring systems have been devised for the trauma patient: (1) Mangled Extremity Severity Score (MESS) and (2) Nerve, Ischemia, Soft Tissue, Skeletal Injury, Shock, Age (NISSSA) score [21,22]. The former looks at limb ischemia, shock, age, and skeletal or soft tissue injury. The latter is more concerned with nerve and soft tissue injury. Both apply numerical values to each characteristic and have threshold scores that indicate a primary amputation.

Postoperatively, if the incision and drainage with the amputation was successful, skin lines of the remaining portion of the foot should reappear in a few days, which signify reduction in edema. Any leukocytosis lessens, cultures at dressing changes are negative, and any general malaise disappears. One also may see the emergence of postinflammatory hyperpigmentation. If the presenting signs and symptoms remain unchanged or a foot beginning to recover takes a turn for the worse, another incision and drainage is planned. More tissue may have to be removed.

Finally, one of the best "tools" in the arsenal of a surgeon is experience. The more one is faced with cases requiring an amputation, the more one is able to discover subtle signs of viability, discuss with ease the possibility of amputation with a patient, and accept the lessened likelihood of taking just a small part and avoid doing too many surgeries on the same patient. Experience also provides one with the ability to look at a foot and decide that the entire lower extremity cannot be saved and a more proximal amputation (below-knee amputation or above-knee amputation) provides the only option.

Other considerations with amputations

In most cases when an amputation is performed, the incisions cited in the literature can be used. These affect primary closure. In some cases, owing to previous tissue loss or ulcerations, incisions have to be creative. Additionally the level of amputation may be more proximal than described in any resource. An example is a diabetic with an ulcer beneath the third metatarsal head that requires a TMA. As a result of the necrotic tissue, the ulcer is incorporated within the plantar incision, which yields, for all intents and purposes, a plantar deficit more proximal at the ulcer site. The incision can be converted easily into a T-shaped incision on closure (Fig. 12).

Is function a concern? When one is dealing with a noninfected or severely traumatized part, performing an amputation at the proper level respects function. In patients with abundant devitalized tissue requiring débridement, especially in the presence of an infection, function is not at the forefront of the decision process. Here the object is to eradicate the infection by incising, draining, and débriding tissue affected by the disease process.

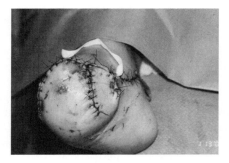

Fig. 12. Plantar ulcer excised within the TMA flap. Note the residual T incision, which was easily closed.

At the closure procedure, the functional aspect of the remaining foot can be addressed and the proper steps taken. The wound edges are excised to bleeding by taking approximately 2 mm of tissue around the entire wound. The flap also is included in this minimal resection. Any bone edges in the wound are resected to healthy bleeding bone. In some instances, this may be only a few more millimeters. The wound is pulsed with irrigation of choice. Drapes, gowns, gloves, and instruments should be changed for the next part of the operation. At that time, any tendon transfers deemed necessary are performed along with the desired method of closure (Fig. 13).

Any surgeon who performs amputations should have, as part of their team, a vascular surgeon, infectious disease physician, and an orthotist/prosthetist. The patient's own primary care physician has to provide the important medical optimization for the patient to undergo this type of surgery.

Although preventing amputations resulting from trauma or a tumor is almost impossible, in a cohort of diabetics, proper education decreased the number of

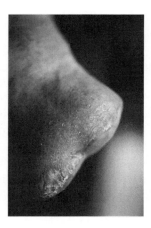

Fig. 13. Proximal forefoot amputation with no tendon transfers performed. Severe varus was evident.

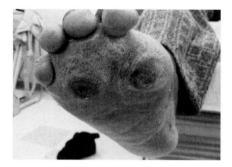

Fig. 14. Preulcerative lesions requiring frequent débridement to prevent further progression.

amputations [23]. Proper foot care and being cognizant of abnormal findings with prompt physician visits should lessen amputations (Fig. 14).

Summary

Amputation may take a psychological toll on a patient. Proper documentation is paramount along with a lucid consent. Various pathologies may lead to an amputation. Tools to aid in the decision to amputate, in choosing the levels of amputation, and in the selection of the type of procedure are available. The key to any amputation is to be at a level that is most definitive.

References

[1] Stedman's Medical Dictionary. 26 edition. Baltimore: Williams & Wilkins; 1995. p. 65.
[2] Shalala DE. Healthy people 2000 midcourse review and 1995 revisions. Washington: US Department of Health and Human Services, Public Health Service; 2000.
[3] Centers for Disease Control and Prevention. The public health of diabetes mellitus in the United States. Atlanta: Department of Health and Human Services; 1997.
[4] Carrington AL, Mawdsley SKV, Morleg M, et al. Psychological status of diabetic people with or without lower limb disability. Diabetes Res Clin Pract 1996;32:19–25.
[5] Bunch W. Informed consent. Clin Orthop 2000;378:71–7.
[6] Lipsky BA. Infectious problems of the foot in diabetic patients. In: Bowker JH, Pfeifer MA, editors. The diabetic foot. 6th edition. St. Louis: Mosby; 2001. p. 467–80.
[7] Lavery LA, Armstrong DG, Quebedeaux TL, Walker SC. Puncture wounds: normal laboratory values in the face of severe infection in diabetics and non-diabetics. Am J Med 1998;101:521–5.
[8] Arroyo CI, Tritto VG, Buchbinder D, et al. Optimal waiting period for limb salvage surgery following limb revascularization. J Foot Ankle Surg 2002;41:228–32.
[9] Pinzur MS, Shields N, Trepman E, Dawson P, Evans A. Current practice patterns in the treatment of Charcot foot. Foot Ankle Int 2000;21:916–20.
[10] Larsen K, Fabian J, Holstein PE. Incidence and management of ulcers in diabetic Charcot feet. J Wound Care 2000;10:320–8.
[11] Akin S. An unusual and nonclassified central polydactyly of the foot. Ann Plast Surg 2004;53: 86–8.

[12] Gustilo RB. Management of open fractures. In: Gustilo RB, Gruninger RP, Tsukayama DT, editors. Orthopaedic infection diagnosis and treatment. Philadelphia: WB Saunders; 1989. p. 87–117.

[13] White CB, Turner NS, Lee GC, Haidukewych GJ. Open ankle fractures in patients with diabetes mellitus. Clin Orthop 2003;414:37–44.

[14] Finley RK, Driscoll DL, Blumenson LE. Subungual melanoma: an eighteen year review. Surgery 1994;116:96–100.

[15] Tice AD, Hoaglund PA, Shoultz DA. Outcomes of osteomyelitis of patients treated with outpatient parental antimicrobial therapy. Am J Med 2003;114:723–8.

[16] Vora AM, Schon LC. Revision peripheral nerve surgery. Foot Ankle Clin N Am 2001;9:305–18.

[17] Wallace GF, Pachuda NM, Gumann G. Open fractures. In: Gumann G, editor. Fractures of the foot and ankle. Philadelphia: WB Saunders; 2004. p. 1–41.

[18] Teodorescu VJ, Chen C, Morrissey N, et al. Detailed protocol of ischemia and the use of non-invasive vascular laboratory testing in diabetic foot ulcers. Am J Surg 2004;187:755–805.

[19] Quigley FG, Faris IB. Trauscutaneous oxygen tension measurements in the assessment of limb ischaemia. Clin Physiol 1991;11:315–20.

[20] Zgonis T, Jolly GP, Buren BJ, Blume P. Diabetic foot infections and antibiotic therapy. Clin Podiatr Med Surg 2003;20:655–69.

[21] Gregory RT, Gould RJ, Peclet M, et al. The mangled extremity syndrome (MES): a severity grading system for multisystem injury of the extremity. J Trauma 1985;25:1147–50.

[22] McNamara MG, Heckman JD, Corley FG. Severe open fractures of the lower extremity: a retrospective evaluation of the mangled extremity severity score (MESS). J Orthop Trauma 1994;8:81–7.

[23] Wrobel JS, Charns MP, Diehr P, et al. The relationship between provider coordination and diabetes-related foot outcomes. Diabetes Care 2003;26:3042–7.

ELSEVIER
SAUNDERS

Clin Podiatr Med Surg
22 (2005) 329–341

CLINICS IN
PODIATRIC
MEDICINE AND
SURGERY

Perioperative Management of Pedal Amputations

Keith D. Cook, DPM

Podiatry Service, University Hospital–University of Medicine and Dentistry of New Jersey,
150 Bergen Street, Room A-226, Newark, NJ 07103, USA

Performing a pedal amputation, whether as a result of infection, trauma, frostbite, peripheral vascular disease, neoplasm, or congenital deformity, always must begin with medical management of the patient. Any amputation has physical and psychological effects on a patient, which need to be addressed and treated accordingly. Proper perioperative management and preoperative planning are essential to any successful surgical procedure. The fact that the amputee may have existing comorbidities accentuates the importance of proper perioperative management.

At the author's institution, a multidisciplinary approach is used in the care of the pedal amputation patient. The team consists of podiatrists, hospitalists, vascular surgeons, radiologists, physical therapists, nutritionists, orthotists, and social workers and cardiologists, nephrologists, and psychiatrists when required. The hospital's medicine consult team comanages every patient admitted to the Podiatry Service. Each patient also has standard tests are performed on admission. These tests consist of baseline laboratory studies and plain radiographs of the affected foot. When vascular compromise is suspected, as is the case in many diabetics, noninvasive vascular studies and a vascular consultation are obtained. In addition, deep vein thrombosis (DVT) prophylaxis is initiated for every patient admitted.

A hospital nutritionist evaluates the patient, and an appropriate diet is started based on the patient's medical and nutritional needs. A proper diet can be essential in optimizing wound healing. If the patient is found to need special services or residence placement when discharged, the social services department is contacted immediately. The social worker enables proper placement of the

E-mail address: cookkd@umdnj.edu

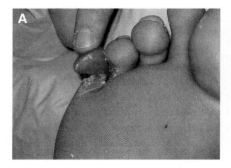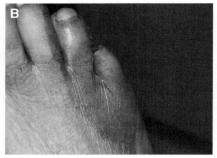

Fig. 1. Patient with a painful fifth digit ainhum. (*A*) Preoperatively. (*B*) Status post partial fifth digit amputation. The patient had immediate relief of pain.

patient and prevents any delays in discharge; this helps to decrease hospital length of stay and medical costs.

All patients who are having an amputation performed as a same-day surgery procedure should follow the protocol of the particular institution. Completion of an autoamputation as a result of an ainhum constriction may be performed as a same-day procedure (Fig. 1). Preoperative testing should consist of the radiographic and laboratory testing that is routinely performed for any podiatric same-day surgical procedure. Medical clearance also should be obtained.

Laboratory workup

Preoperative laboratory studies should be performed on all patients requiring an amputation. This screening consists of a complete blood count with differential, complete metabolic panel, prothrombin time, and partial thromboplastin time. The complete blood count with differential is essential to determine if an infectious process is occurring. An elevated white blood cell count (>12,000 cells/mm^3) and an increase in polymorphonuclear leukocytes indicate an acute infection. The white blood cell count and polymorphonuclear leukocytes may not be elevated, however, in the presence of infection in an immunocompromised host, such as a diabetic or patient with AIDS. A low hemoglobin and hematocrit, if noted in the complete blood count with differential, may attribute to poor tissue oxygenation and decreased healing potential. Any abnormalities should be addressed accordingly.

The complete metabolic panel consists of electrolytes, blood urea nitrogen, serum creatinine, glucose levels, and liver function tests. The electrolytes, blood urea nitrogen, and serum creatinine levels are essential in assessing hydration and the status of the patient's renal function. Intravenous fluids and medications including antibiotics may need to be adjusted based on these results. If the patient's renal function is impaired, a renal consultation should be obtained. Any patient who receives hemodialysis should be maintained on their normal schedule. The surgical procedure should be performed on an alternating day when the patient does not receive dialysis.

Liver function tests, including bilirubin, albumin, total protein, aspartate aminotransferase, and alanine aminotransferase levels, help to determine if any hepatic disease is present in which certain medications may need to be adjusted. The presence of hepatic disease or decrease in liver function may impede wound healing.

Serum glucose levels commonly are elevated in a diabetic patient in the presence of infection. Hemoglobin A_{1C} level should be obtained to assess the long-term glucose control of the diabetic patient. If osteomyelitis is suspected, erythrocyte sedimentation rate and C-reactive protein tests also are ordered. These tests are nonspecific but sensitive for an inflammatory process.

Cardiac evaluation

At the author's institution, all patients older than age 40 or with a history of cardiac disease have a 12-lead ECG performed preoperatively. When indicated, patients also receive an echocardiogram and evaluation by the cardiology team. Further testing, including cardiac catheterization, is performed as needed. In these patients, cardiology clearance for anesthesia is required before any surgical intervention.

Vascular evaluation

The lower extremity vascular status of any patient should never be assumed or taken for granted. A full lower extremity vascular examination beginning with palpation of pulses should be performed. If the pulses are nonpalpable or other signs of vascular insufficiency are present, such as atrophic skin changes and loss of digital hair, a bedside arterial Doppler examination is conducted. Evaluation for monophasic, biphasic, or triphasic arterial Doppler signals helps in determining the arterial circulatory status. Triphasic or biphasic Doppler signals are consistent with healthy vessels, whereas monophasic signals indicate arterial occlusive disease with decreased blood flow.

For most amputee patients, especially diabetics, noninvasive vascular studies are essential in determining healing potential and level of amputation. Measurement of arterial pressures, ankle-brachial index (ABI), and pulse volume recordings is performed routinely at the author's institution (Fig. 2). Although ABIs may be falsely elevated secondary to arterial wall calcification and noncompressibility of the vessels, some authors have shown that they are as valuable as other diagnostic studies in the clinical outcome of critical limb ischemia [1]. ABIs are less beneficial, however, in determining the level of arterial disease or occlusion. Further diagnostic studies are required.

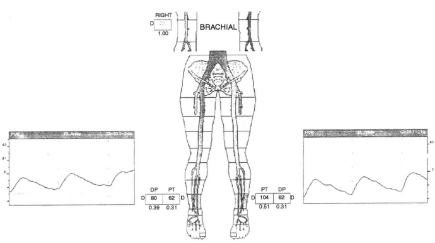

Fig. 2. Noninvasive arterial studies of a patient with dry gangrene of her right foot fifth digit. Her right side ABI was 0.31 with poor pulse volume recordings. A partial fifth ray amputation was performed 4 days after lower extremity angioplasty was performed by the vascular surgery team at the author's institution.

Transcutaneous oxygen pressures, skin thermography, skin blood flow, and skin perfusion pressures have been shown to be more effective in determining proper amputation levels and preventing reamputation [2–5]. These studies provide a more accurate level of ischemia and predictive value of healing. A study conducted by the Vascular Surgery Department at the author's institution proved that transcutaneous oxygen pressure studies, with 83% accuracy, are superior to segmental pressures or ABIs when estimating the probability of healing [6]. Misuri et al [2] determined a threshold of 20 mm Hg with transcutaneous oximetry when determining amputation level. Any transcutaneous oxygen pressure reading less than 20 mm Hg is a poor indicator for healing, and a more proximal amputation may need to be considered, unless revascularization or increased perfusion can be achieved.

When the aforementioned tests indicate poor healing potential, except in the emergent situation, a vascular surgery consultation is obtained, and further diagnostic studies are performed. The vascular surgery team can order digital subtraction angiography, carbon dioxide angiography, magnetic resonance arteriography, or spiral CT angiography to help determine the level of arterial occlusive disease and surgical planning. "Contrast angiography remains the gold standard in diagnostic studies upon which a treatment plan is formulated" [7]. Should a blockage be discovered, various types of intervention, including endarterectomy, balloon angioplasty, or bypass reconstruction, may be employed to increase perfusion and decrease the chance of a more proximal amputation. In some instances, a combination of procedures may need to be performed. Only after successful revascularization of an ischemic limb should a definitive amputation be scheduled. No amputation is performed for at least 72 hours after bypass revascularization [8].

Deep vein thrombosis prophylaxis

The incidence of DVT has been well documented after general and orthopedic surgery. Patients undergoing lower extremity amputation are considered to be at a high risk for DVT. Studies have shown the incidence of DVT in patients who undergo lower extremity amputations to be 12.5% to 50% [9–11].

Virchow's triad of stasis, blood vessel injury, and hypercoagulability is experienced to some degree by an amputation patient regardless of the indication for or level of amputation. The patient undergoing an amputation is at an increased risk for developing a DVT, and proper prophylactic measures need to be instituted. Standard DVT prophylaxis consists of subcutaneous injections of low-dose unfractionated heparin or low-molecular-weight heparin. If a DVT is suspected, appropriate diagnostic venous duplex studies should be performed immediately, and, if positive, appropriate DVT treatment should be initiated without delay.

The DVT prophylaxis protocol followed by the Podiatry Service at the author's institution consists of 30 mg of enoxaparin administered subcutaneously every 12 hours, initiated on admission. The enoxaparin is held 12 hours before surgery and restarted 12 hours postoperatively. Antiembolism stockings are applied to the contralateral limb at the time of surgery and are worn throughout the patient's hospitalization. Early postoperative mobilization and weight bearing when appropriate are initiated with assistance from the physical therapy department. The patients also are encouraged to be out of bed and sit upright in a chair.

Antibiotics

The use of antibiotics is not always necessary when performing a pedal amputation. The indication for the amputation and medical status of the patient are the driving forces for the surgeon to decide if and what type of antibiotic therapy is necessary.

Most traumatic amputations are considered to be open fractures and follow the guidelines for open fracture treatment. The protocol followed by the Podiatry Service at the author's institution consists of immediate surgical débridement and pulse lavage followed by 72 hours of intravenous antibiotics. The antibiotics consist of a first-generation cephalosporin and an aminoglycoside. The author uses cefazolin, 2 g initially followed by 1 g every 8 hours, and gentamicin, 5 mg/kg once daily. If the injury is contaminated with grass or soil, such as from a lawn mower injury (Fig. 3), 10 to 20 million U of penicillin are given daily in divided

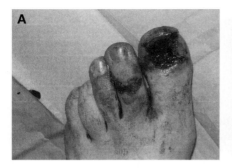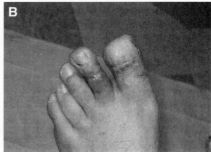

Fig. 3. Patient who sustained a lawn mower injury to his left foot. (*A*) Preoperatively. (*B*) 2 months postoperatively. The second digit was salvageable, whereas a distal Symes amputation was required for the hallux.

doses [12]. The cephalosporin may be substituted with clindamycin for patients with a penicillin allergy.

Patients who undergo pedal amputations as a result of an infectious process are started on a broad-spectrum antibiotic, such as pipercillin-tazobactam or ampicillin-sulbactam. The antibiotics are not a substitute for urgent operative incision and drainage, however. Intraoperative cultures of the amputation site are obtained after pulse lavage. The wound is packed open. At the first dressing change, 36 to 48 hours postoperatively, a new set of cultures is obtained. The antibiotic may be changed then, if no clinical signs of improvement are evident, to one with a more narrow-spectrum sensitive to any existing organisms obtained from the two cultures. The patient is brought back to the operating room for additional débridement and irrigation as needed. The wound is closed after a clean culture is obtained, and the wound is granular, the edema is minimal, and there is no leukocytosis.

If a dead space is maintained on final closure of the wound, the space may be occupied with antibiotic beads. Resorbable calcium sulfate or calcium phosphate beads impregnated with vancomycin or tobramycin are used. The resorbable

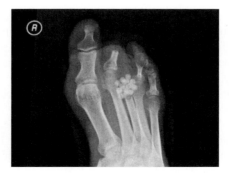

Fig. 4. Patient status post partial second toe and partial third ray amputation, secondary to wet gangrene. The dead space was filled with tobramycin-impregnated calcium sulfate beads.

beads elude antibiotics locally into the wound and prevent hematoma formation. The fact the beads resorb eliminates the need for removal (Fig. 4).

Imaging modalities

Various imaging modalities are available to evaluate the prospective pedal amputee, each with specific advantages and disadvantages. The proper modality for evaluation must be chosen based on the indication for the amputation and should aid in the assessment of amputation level.

All patients initially obtain plain film radiographs. Plain film radiographs are useful in evaluating the types of fractures involved in the trauma patient and if reconstruction is possible. Initial radiographs also may reveal bony involvement of neoplasms, congenital abnormalities, infectious processes, and the presence of gas in the soft tissue (Fig. 5). More specific testing should be performed, however, as each situation warrants establishing a diagnosis and determining the appropriate level of amputation.

CT scans have been used to detect bone sequestra, cortical destruction, and periosteal new bone formation [13]. CT scans also are useful in diagnosing bone tumors, occult fractures, and abscess formation. CT scans combined with contrast administration are ordered to diagnose abscess formation. CT is inferior to MRI, however, in diagnosing soft tissue neoplasms or osteomyelitis. MRI helps in determining the extent of neoplastic or infectious involvement and may yield insight to the proper level of amputation. MRI may fall short in differentiating between osteomyelitis and neuroarthropathy [14].

Nuclear scans are more effective than MRI in differentiating between osteomyelitis and neuroarthropathy and a variety of other pathologies. Each type of nuclear study has advantages and disadvantages. Technetium-99m (^{99m}Tc) scans have a high sensitivity and a low specificity when evaluating bone pa-

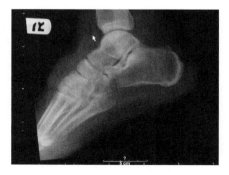

Fig. 5. Patient with a fetid foot and radiographic evidence of gas gangrene along the dorsal aspect of the foot. Arrow points to gas tracking up the patient's leg and separation of the tissue planes. This resulted in a below-knee amputation.

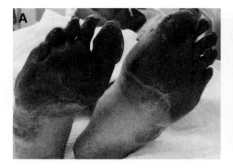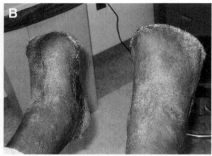

Fig. 6. Patient with bilateral forefoot frostbite. (*A*) Preoperatively. (*B*) 6 weeks status post bilateral transmetatarsal amputations.

thology. They are useful for evaluating occult fractures and have been used to assess soft tissue perfusion and level of amputation required for patients with frostbite (Fig. 6) [15].

Various other nuclear imaging modalities are available to the foot and ankle surgeon to determine the appropriate level of amputation or limb salvage, including indium-111 (^{111}In)-oxine, ^{99m}Tc-HMPAO, ^{99m}Tc–stannous fluoride colloid labeled leukocytes, and gallium-67 (^{67}Ga)-citrate scans. Each of these nuclear studies has specific advantages and disadvantages in diagnosing different infectious processes (Table 1). It is beyond the scope of this article to describe each scan in detail; however, their radiopharmaceutical properties need to be understood and the proper study chosen to diagnose osteomyelitis versus

Table 1
Nuclear imaging modalities

Nuclear imaging modalities	Advantages	Disadvantages
[111]In-oxine	Normal constant biodistribution	Can accumulate in sites of inflammation without infection
	High sensitivity for osteomyelitis	Does not detect viral or paracytic infections
^{99m}Tc-HMPAO	Cheaper than ^{111}In-oxine	Poor distribution
	Improved visualization in feet	Does not detect viral or paracytic infections
	Localizes in infectious sites rapidly	
[99m]Tc–stannous flouride colloid	Inexpensive	Inferior sensitivity and specificity compared with ^{111}In-oxine
	Non–labor intensive procedure	
[67]Ga-citrate	Low toxicity	Low specificity
	Can detect bacterial and nonbacterial infections	

Table 2
Nuclear imaging indications

Pathology	Nuclear study
Soft tissue infection	^{99m}Tc-HMPAO
Abscess	^{111}In-oxine
Acute osteomyelitis	^{99m}Tc-HMPAO
Chronic osteomyelitis	^{111}In-oxine plus
	^{99m}Tc–stannous flouride colloid
Occult fever	^{111}In-oxine

neuroarthropathy or soft tissue infection (Table 2) [16]. Limb salvage surgical planning can then proceed.

Informed consent

Obtaining surgical consent for an amputation is difficult for the patient and the surgeon. The surgeon must explain to the patient in layman's terms the way he or she is going to remove part of their limb, along with the expected postoperative course. Depending on the circumstances or reason for the amputation (eg, an infectious process), the patient must be made to understand that more than one trip to the operating room and revision of the original procedure may be required. At the author's institution, consent always is obtained from amputation patients for a more proximal amputation than what is anticipated. The patient also gives consent for removal of all necrotic, infected, or nonsalvageable bone, skin, and soft tissue. Even with the best surgical planning and preoperative testing, unforeseen circumstances still can occur in the operating room. The ability to amend the original anticipated surgical procedure intraoperatively may be necessary despite preoperative preparation.

Psychological ramifications

The old adage "the foot is attached to the rest of the body" is never more accurate than when part or all of that foot is going to be removed. Amputation of a body part, whether as a result of trauma, peripheral vascular disease, frostbite, infection, or neoplasm, has psychological effects on the patient. Although some patients may be relieved after removing a painful limb, most amputation procedures have an adverse psychological effect on patients. In a study by Refaat et al [17], comparison of psychological issues between patients with amputations and patients with limb-sparing procedures for extremity sarcomas revealed that 26% of the amputees studied had depression, 26% had anxiety, and 38% had sleep disturbances. These findings were not statistically significant, however, compared with the limb-sparing group.

A complication of an amputation that should be treated by multiple disciplines is phantom limb pain. Phantom limb pain is defined as painful sensations in the amputated limb [18]. In a study conducted by van der Schans et al [18], patients who experienced phantom limb pain had a poorer health-related quality of life than amputees without phantom limb pain. When a patient experiences phantom limb pain, he or she should be referred immediately to a psychiatrist and a pain management physician so that treatment can be rendered from multiple disciplines with a focus to improve the patient's quality of life. Physical therapy also should be initiated as early as the healing amputation allows.

When patients are having difficulty coping with their amputation, a psychiatry or bereavement counselor consultation is obtained. Counseling is begun while the patient is still admitted and continues in the outpatient setting as necessary. For some patients, the psychological ramifications of an amputation are more difficult to "heal" than the actual surgical procedure.

Hospital discharge

The amputee patient under the care of the Podiatry Service at the author's institution is discharged only after a definitive procedure has been performed. Ideally the amputation site should be closed either primarily or with a skin flap or graft. If a wound is to be closed via secondary intention, local wound care is performed by the patient on discharge, or arrangements are made to include a visiting health care professional. All discharges are coordinated with the social services department. The patient also must be cleared for discharge by all of the consultation teams treating the patient.

When an amputation is performed secondary to an infectious process, it is assumed that all osteomyelitis has been removed. It is not essential for the patient to continue intravenous antibiotic treatment. On discharge at the author's institution, the Podiatry Service protocol is to convert the patient to oral antibiotics for 2 weeks. The amputee patient is followed on a weekly basis at the Podiatry Center. If the wound develops a superficial infection during the course of antibiotics, the antibiotic is switched to an agent that is sensitive to any existing organisms. If a limb-threatening infection redevelops, the patient is readmitted for intravenous antibiotic therapy and incision and drainage.

On successful wound healing, the staples or sutures that were used for wound closure are removed. These are removed usually 2 to 3 weeks postoperatively. The rehabilitation process then proceeds.

Rehabilitation

After an amputation has healed, the patient must learn how to ambulate and perform activities of daily living without part of the lower extremity. This process is started while the patient is in the hospital and as early in the recovery period as possible. Patients are instructed to begin ambulation on the first postoperative day. Partial–weight-bearing or non–weight-bearing gait training, depending on the patient's medical condition and amputation level, is conducted by a physical therapist. The patient is not discharged until the physical therapist determines that the patient can ambulate safely with crutches, walker, or other assistive device; this is documented in the patient's chart.

It has been well researched that a more proximal lower extremity amputation increases energy expenditure. Studies also have shown that patients with distal amputations have a greater independence and less impairment compared with their counterparts with amputations at a more proximal level [19–21]. These facts must be remembered when planning the amputation procedure. The most distal amputation possible should be performed to expedite recovery and decrease morbidity.

Proper tendon balancing and appropriate biomechanical considerations also must be taken into account when performing an amputation for the patient to fit into a prosthesis or custom shoe. If the biomechanics of the foot are ignored, residual deformities in the sagittal, frontal, and transverse planes may occur, which result in an inability to wear a prosthesis properly, increased impairment, and possibly further amputation. Patients are more functional with distal amputations and properly maintained biomechanics [19].

A retrospective study conducted by Pezzin et al [22] showed that patients who are fitted for a prosthesis in a shorter time frame after their amputation were more likely to use the device and had a greater satisfaction rate with the prosthesis. The patient should be fitted for a prosthesis, custom-made shoe, or brace as soon as the amputation site has healed completely. Prostheses also improve the gait pattern of the amputee, even with distal pedal amputations [23].

The Podiatry Center at the author's institution works closely with certified orthotists and pedorthists. The amputation patient is evaluated in conjunction with the orthotist to determine the appropriate prosthesis and custom-made shoe to optimize patient function and activity. The patient is followed on a regular basis after receiving the device, and modifications are made as deemed necessary.

Summary

The perioperative management of an amputation patient is a multidisciplinary task. Regardless of the indication for the amputation, proper surgical planning, including radiographic, vascular, and laboratory studies, is needed. The patient needs to be medically optimized for the surgical procedure, and consultation with other services needs to be obtained when warranted. If vascular compromise is present, revascularization by a vascular surgeon should be attempted.

When treating an amputation patient, it is important to manage the psychological effects the amputation may have on the patient as well as the surgical procedure itself. If necessary, a psychiatry consultation should be obtained. It has been reported that patients with distal amputations have a better quality of life and less morbidity than patients with more proximal amputations. After proper preoperative planning, the most distal amputation that would heal properly should be performed.

The surgeon also must understand the biomechanics of the foot when performing an amputation with proper skin closure and tendon balancing to prevent further pedal deformity and complications. The foot and ankle surgeon should work closely with an orthotist, have the patient fitted for a prosthesis as soon as healing allows, and follow the patient regularly for any prosthetic modifications that are needed.

The foot and ankle surgeon needs to manage the amputation patient effectively preoperatively, intraoperatively, and postoperatively to achieve an optimal surgical outcome. This management enables proper healing, decreased morbidity, and quick return to daily activities for the patient.

References

[1] de Graff J, Ubbink D, Legemate D, Tijssen J, Jacobs M. Evaluation of toe pressure and transcutaneous oxygen measurements in management of chronic critical leg ischemia: a diagnostic randomized clinical trial. J Vasc Surg 2003;38:528–34.

[2] Misuri A, Lucertini G, Nanni A, Viacava A, Belardi P. Predictive value of transcutaneous oximetry for selection of the amputation level. J Cardiovasc Surg (Torino) 2000;41:83–7.

[3] Ohsawa S, Inamori Y, Fukuda K, Hirotuji M. Lower limb amputation for diabetic foot. Arch Orthop Trauma Surg 2001;121:186–90.

[4] Welch G, Leiberman D, Pollock J, Angerson W. Failure of Doppler ankle pressure to predict healing of conservative forefoot amputations. Br J Surg 1985;72:888–91.

[5] Castronuovo J, Adera H, Smiell J, Price R. Skin perfusion pressure measurement is valuable in the diagnosis of critical limb ischemia. J Vasc Surg 1997;26:629–37.

[6] Padberg F, Back T, Thompson P, Hobson R. Transcutaneous oxygen (TcPo$_2$) estimates probability of healing in the ischemic extremity. J Surg Res 1996;60:365–9.

[7] Andros G. Diagnostic and therapeutic arterial interventions in the ulcerated diabetic foot. Diabetes Metab Res Rev 2004;20(Suppl 1):S29–33.

[8] Arroyo C, Tritto V, Buchbinder D, et al. Optimal waiting period for foot salvage surgery following limb revascularization. J Foot Ankle Surg 2002;41:228–32.

[9] Yeager R, Moneta G, Edwards J, Taylor L, McConnell D, Porter J. Deep vein thrombosis associated with lower extremity amputation. J Vasc Surg 1995;22:612–5.

[10] Fletcher J, Batiste P. Incidence of deep vein thrombosis following vascular surgery. Int Angiol 1997;16:65–8.

[11] Burke B, Kumar R, Vickers V, Grant E, Scremin E. Deep vein thrombosis after lower limb amputation. Am J Phys Med Rehabil 2000;79:145–9.

[12] Healey K, Danis K. Treatment of open fractures. Clin Podiatr Med Surg 1995;12:791–800.

[13] Sella E, Grosser D. Imaging modalities of the diabetic foot. Clin Podiatr Med Surg 2003;20:729–40.

[14] Seabold J, Flickinger F, Simon C. Indium-111-leukocyte/technetium-99m-MDP bone and magnetic resonance imaging: difficulty of diagnosing osteomyelitis in patients with neuropathic osteoarthropathy. J Nucl Med 1990;31:549–56.

[15] Aygit A, Sarikaya A. Imaging of frostbite injury by technetium-99m-sestamibi scintigraphy: a case report. Foot Ankle Int 2002;23:56–9.

[16] Hughes D. Nuclear medicine and infection detection: the relative effectiveness of imaging with

111In-oxine-, 99m-Tc-HMPAO-, and 99m-Tc-stannous fluoride colloid-labeled leukocytes and with 67Ga-citrate. J Nucl Med Technol 2003;31:196–201.

[17] Refaat Y, Gunnoe J, Hornicek F, Mankin H. Comparison of quality of life after amputation or limb salvage. Clin Orthop 2002;397:298–305.

[18] van der Schans C, Geertzen J, Schoppen T, Dijkstra P. Phantom pain and health-related quality of life in lower limb amputees. J Pain Symptom Manage 2002;24:429–36.

[19] Davis B, Kuznicki J, Praveen S, Sferra J. Lower-extremity amputations in patients with diabetes: pre- and post-surgical decisions related to successful rehabilitation. Diabetes Metab Res Rev 2004;20(Suppl 1):S45–50.

[20] Franchignoni F, Orlandini D, Ferriero G, Moscato T. Reliability, validity, and responsiveness of the locomotor capabilities index in adults with lower-limb amputation undergoing prosthetic training. Arch Phys Med Rehabil 2004;85:743–8.

[21] Peters E, Childs M, Wunderlich R, Harkless L, Armstrong D, Lavery L. Functional status of persons with diabetes-related lower-extremity amputations. Diabetes Care 2001;24:1799–804.

[22] Pezzin L, Dillingham T, MacKenzie E, Ephraim P, Rossbach P. Use and satisfaction with prosthetic limb devices and related services. Arch Phys Med Rehabil 2004;85:723–9.

[23] Tang S, Chen C, Chen M, Chen W, Leong C, Chu N. Transmetatarsal amputation prosthesis with carbon-fiber plate: enhanced gait function. Am J Phys Med Rehabil 2004;83(2):124–30.

ELSEVIER
SAUNDERS

Clin Podiatr Med Surg
22 (2005) 343–363

CLINICS IN
PODIATRIC
MEDICINE AND
SURGERY

Digital Amputations

Ritchard C. Rosen, DPM, FACFAS, FAPWCA[a,b,c,*]

[a]*Podiatric Surgery, Holy Name Hospital, 718 Teaneck Road, Teaneck, NJ 07666, USA*
[b]*University Hospital–University of Medicine and Dentistry of New Jersey, PO Box 1709,
Newark, NJ 07101, USA*
[c]*American Board of Podiatric Surgery, 445 Fillmore Street, San Francisco, CA 94117-3404, USA*

In the past, partial foot amputations—and more specifically, digital amputations, defined in this article as amputations at the metatarsophalangeal joint or any level distal to this joint—were performed almost exclusively for trauma. As a result of advances in vascular reconstruction, broader spectrum antibiotics, the accepted use of local anesthesia, and an interdisciplinary approach to the patient with foot pathology, however, digital amputations have become more popular. Once considered a crude, mundane procedure, amputation should be viewed in the same light as other reconstructive and elective procedures. The results of digital amputations have improved greatly with these measures, and if complications arise, minimal time, cost, and risk have been lost. Other advances that have assisted the success of distal amputations include proper nutrition, wound healing centers, strict protocols of wound healing, and the advent of hyperbaric oxygen chambers.

Amputation often arises in emergent situations as a result of infection, ischemia, or trauma. Digital amputations also may be performed to correct congenital anomalies, such as polydactylism, and for removal of malignant tumors.

The psychologic and biomechanic aspects of digital amputation must be kept in mind because it is a loss of a body part, however small, to the patient. Amputation should be viewed as an attempt to heal and allow the patient to resume a more normal daily existence without disease. With proper clinical assessment, patient and family education, appropriate surgical procedure, postoperative care, adequate follow-up, rehabilitation, and shoe modifications as

* 142 Engle Street, Englewood, NJ 07631.
E-mail address: R-Rosen@mail.holyname.org

0891-8422/05/$ – see front matter © 2005 Elsevier Inc. All rights reserved.
doi:10.1016/j.cpm.2005.03.001
podiatric.theclinics.com

necessary, the surgeon and patient should be able to attain the goal of resumed normal function.

This article takes a closer look at the reasons for amputation and procedures indicated for each. Amputation should be considered not a failure, but a way for patients to return to normal activity. Each surgeon has his or her preference as to specific incisions for digital amputation, but the more common procedures are highlighted.

The diabetic foot is a major cause of morbidity and mortality, with a 50% to 70% major lower extremity amputation rate [1]. Untreated diabetic foot ulcerations lead to an 84% risk for amputation. Diabetic foot ulcers are 62% neuropathic, 13% vascular, and 28% combined [2]. The most common cause of digital amputation is wet gangrene caused by infection. Most digital amputations occur in patients 45 years of age or younger [3].

The 3-year survival rate in patients who have diabetes mellitus with lower extremity amputations is 50% [4]. The best treatment ultimately is prevention of ulceration and limb-threatening infection. Current studies have demonstrated that regular pedal care may lessen the ill effects of peripheral vascular disease to the foot [5].

Dry gangrene from shower emboli and collagen vascular diseases leading to amputation occurs much less frequently. In the trauma patient, the leading cause of digital amputation is from lawnmower or motorcycle accidents. Thermal injuries (eg, frostbite and burns) also can be a cause for performing digital amputations, whereas tumors of the digits requiring amputation are rare. Regardless of the reason for amputation, care should be taken to plan adequate closure and preservation of skin. The level of amputation should be proximal to the disease process with care taken to remove sharp bone edges and lessen tension on the skin from inadequate bone resections.

The author prefers to be aggressive in the prophylactic treatment of foot lesions in an attempt to prevent amputation. This may include early surgical intervention for hammertoes and other forefoot pathology.

Indications for amputation

General indications for amputation include Trauma, tumor, and transplantation; Infection; Peripheral vascular disease; Congenital deformities (TIPC); chronic pain; electively for deformities in the elderly population; and ingrowing toenails (Box 1) [6]. Specific indications for digital amputations include an ankle-brachial index (ABI) greater than 0.45 [7]; well-demarcated necrosis; no ascending cellulitis, osteomyelitis of the proximal, middle, or distal phalanx; a tumor in the distal half of the digit; symptomatic and cosmetic polydactyly; and donor harvesting for transplantation of the toe to a hand. The absence of pedal pulses is not an indicator of success in amputations [8], but a palpable posterior tibial pulse is associated with 90% healing [9]. If toe pressures are less than 30 mm Hg, critical ischemia is evident and healing problematic [10].

Box 1. General indications for amputation (TIPC)

T: Trauma, tumor, transplantation
I: Infection
P: Peripheral vascular disease
C: Congenital deformities

(*From* Kominsky S. Medical and surgical management of the diabetic foot. St. Louis (MO): C.V. Mosby; 1994; with permission.)

Transcutaneous oxygen measurements are a valuable tool in assessing tissue viability [11–13]. Tissue oxygen levels less than 40 mm Hg also are suggestive of ischemia [10]. Skin quality, temperature, and intraoperative bleeding are also good predictors of healing [14].

Diabetes mellitus with secondary complications of neuropathy and vasculopathy is the most common cause of digital amputation. Simple gangrene with a well-perfused foot will require an amputation of the hallux or digit. One should be cautious because 40% of patients who have diabetes mellitus who undergo minor amputations with well-perfused feet on noninvasive vascular testing will achieve healing, and 20% will undergo a more major proximal amputation [15].

Patients who have gangrene isolated to a digit with an ischemic foot will require revascularization before distal amputation. Postbypass, it is best to wait at least 72 hours before digital amputation to allow for revascularization of ischemic tissue [16].

Trauma is the second-leading cause of digital amputation and the most common cause in the young patient. The most common traumatic causes of amputation are lawnmower and motorcycle injuries. Figs. 1–3 show traumatic injury in a 16-year-old boy who was running in his backyard barefoot. The

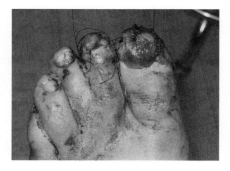

Fig. 1. Closure of lawnmower injury after amputation of tufts of the hallux and second toe.

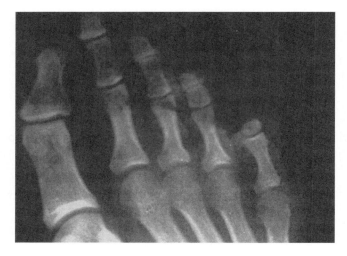

Fig. 2. Preoperative radiograph of severed fifth toe.

patient ran into a steel ladder and sustained a traumatic amputation of his fifth digit through the level of the middle phalanx. Upon presentation to the emergency department, the distal aspect of the digit was absent and brought in ice. Radiographs revealed a clean traumatic amputation through the middle phalanx. It was determined that the distal stump could not be reattached, and the patient was brought to the operating room for debridement and irrigation with 3 L

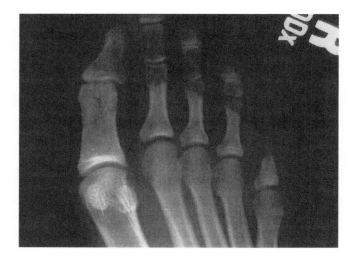

Fig. 3. Final result after irrigation, debridement, and proximal resection.

of saline with cefazolin. Primary closure was performed after a clean resection through the proximal phalanx. The child was placed on ofloxacin and metranidazole and discharged within 24 hours. The patient was seen at 1 and 2 weeks postoperatively, at which time sutures were removed. The child then was instructed to resume a more normal activity level. At 3 months postamputation, the child was healed completely and returned to all levels of activity.

Multiple scoring systems for predicting limb salvage have been described in the literature, including the mangled extremity severity score (MESS) [17]. The MESS, classically for major trauma, may be extrapolated to digital trauma in cases of neurovascular damage from low energy injuries. Higher energy injuries that may cause a pulseless foot and major neurologic injuries would lead to more extensive injuries and probably necessitate a more proximal amputation. It always should be remembered that classifications and scoring systems are guidelines and cannot replace good clinical judgment.

Also included in the trauma category are thermal injuries such as frostbite and burns. (Fig. 4). Electrical burns are complex because the full extent of the injury is not apparent at the initial presentation. Treatment of burns involves early debridement of all devitalized tissue and aggressive treatment. In digital cases, often a primary amputation is a more sensible approach to potential multiple procedures. Frostbite is defined as freezing of tissue. The first step in the treatment of frostbite is to rewarm rapidly the digits in water baths of 104 to 111°F. Blebs developed from the injury should be left intact to minimize infection. Low-dose aspirin or ibuprofen should be administered. In the case of frostbite, in contrast to trauma, burns, and electrical injuries, amputation should be delayed 2 to 6 months to allow devitalized tissue to demarcate. This will minimize unnecessary tissue resection and proximal amputations.

In the treatment of lawnmower and motorcycle injuries, prompt debridement is critical (Fig. 5). The wounds must be debrided and all foreign bodies removed. These amputations must be left open and should be staged, because further necrosis of the skin may occur. Appropriate antibiosis and strict adherence to Gustilo and Anderson's open wound classification must be followed [18].

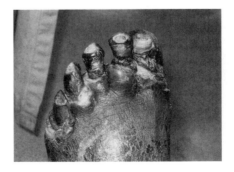

Fig. 4. Digital frostbite.

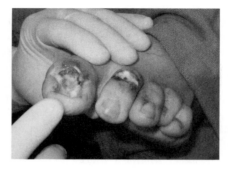

Fig. 5. Appearance of hallux and second toe after irrigation, debridement, and resection of non-viable bone.

Avulsions, degloving, and crush injuries carry a poor prognosis and can lead to digital amputation.

Tumors also may lead to digital amputation. If there is suspicion of malignancy, a more extensive examination with adjunctive procedures is performed. Laboratory studies, standard films, and MRI may be necessary to formulate a differential diagnosis. Additionally, consultation with internal medicine and oncology should be sought in any suspected malignancy. Biopsy is the criterion standard for the definitive diagnosis of any suspicious bone or soft tissue tumor. When performing biopsies on tumors, one must keep in mind that contamination of the unaffected tissues should not occur. In this patient population it is crucial to resect the tumor in its entirety and follow specific protocol for preventing the seeding of malignant cells. Enneking [19] described the concept of surgical margins with reference to various excisional and amputation techniques. Benign tumors rarely require amputation for definitive therapy [20], unless the tumor is so large that resection would compromise the viability of the toe (Fig. 6).

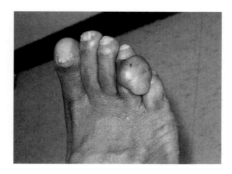

Fig. 6. Extent of tumor necessitated toe amputation.

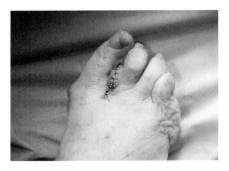

Fig. 7. Amputation of second toe in elderly patient with rigid hammer digit deformity. This is in lieu of forefoot reconstruction.

Congenital deformities such as polydactyly, macrodactyly, and brachymetatarsia also may require digital amputation. The patient may present with dysfunctional digits, and reconstruction may not be a viable treatment option. Also included in these situations of dysfunctional digits are patients who have undergone procedures in which the base of the proximal phalanx has been resected. Although the hammertoe deformity may be corrected, a flail digit may result and cause the patient an unsightly deformity, a painful digit, or difficulty wearing shoes or socks. These patients may benefit greatly from a revisional digital amputation.

Elective amputations of the digits play an important role in the elderly population with severe digital deformities. Patients presenting with severe hallux valgus and second metatarsophalangeal joint dislocations with pain may be better served by an amputation of the second digit rather than reconstruction of the forefoot. The patient will recover more rapidly with fewer potential complications. This patient population will resume normal painfree activity in a timely fashion without prolonged disability. Although a radical approach, the author

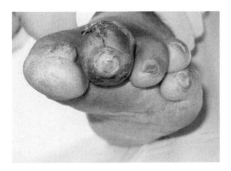

Fig. 8. Exposed distal phalanx at ulcer site.

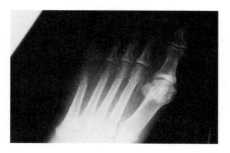

Fig. 9. Chronic osteomyelitis of fifth toe and metatarsal head.

finds that patients are pleased with the final results and return to normal activity in conventional shoes without pain (Fig. 7).

Infection can be a cause of digital amputation in the diabetic, ischemic, or traumatic patient. With digital infections it is of utmost importance to ascertain whether the infection has invaded bone or just the skin and soft tissues. If bone is exposed, one must consider the diagnosis of osteomyelitis (Fig. 8). Radiographs, bone scans, and MRI may be helpful in the diagnosis and assist in the formal level of amputation (Figs. 9–11).

In cases of acute purulent infections, an open amputation is required. This usually is staged and further tissue destruction may occur (Fig. 12). In wounds that are visually clean and the infection is well contained in the structures, however, primary closure may be performed (Fig. 13). An example may be in the situation of osteomyelitis of the distal phalanx secondary to ulceration at the tuft of the digit. If the skin structures are viable and no evidence of proximal infection is apparent, amputation through the proximal phalanx may be performed and closed primarily. Premature closure of infected wounds may lead to a 30% to 40% complication rate (Fig. 14). The advantage of digital amputation over

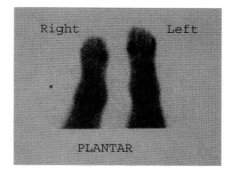

Fig. 10. Bone scan with increased uptake fifth toe left suggestive of osteomyelitis.

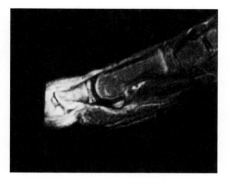

Fig. 11. MRI changes of hallux suggestive of osteomyelitis.

proximal amputation in the foot is that a prosthesis may not be required and the integrity of the lower extremity musculature is maintained, eliminating the necessity of performing additional soft tissue and or tendon transfers.

General principles of amputation

There is no definitive level of surgery in treating specific disease states requiring amputation. The surgeon must be aggressive enough to resect adequately the diseased tissue. In dealing with infection, the primary concern is controlling the systemic infection. The second is to optimize blood flow, then control local

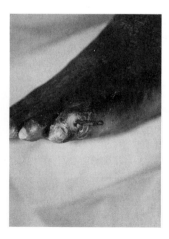

Fig. 12. Purulence from ulcer. The toe was not salvageable.

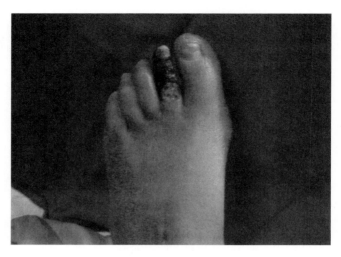

Fig. 13. Gangrene of distal second toe.

infection and achieve a healthy wound. The last important concern is to perform a biomechanically stable amputation [10].

The initial questions to be answered when dealing with digital amputations are: (1) disarticulation or resection through bone, and (2) is it appropriate to leave articular cartilage or should it be resected?

Bowker [21] stated that the articular cartilage should be resected because it is no longer perfused. Moore and Jolly [22] believe that all cartilage should be denuded to avoid subsequent necrosis and formation of draining sinus tracts. These positions may be valid histologically and microscopically, but in practice, cartilage often is left intact as a barrier for infection. Denuding cartilage will expose the medullary canal and allow for potential proximal migration of bac-

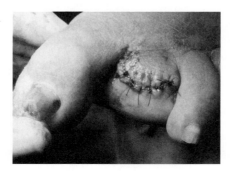

Fig. 14. Drainage from medial aspect of wound after premature closure of the amputation site.

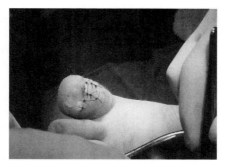

Fig. 15. Modified distal Symes amputation closed 5 days after initial incision and drainage.

teria. When the infectious process is well contained and distal to the joint level, disarticulation with the cartilage intact is appropriate. If tension is present at the wound edges or an open amputation is perfomed, however, the author resects cartilage and follows strict wound-care protocols before formal closure.

The second decision a surgeon must make at the time of surgery is whether to close the wound primarily or to stage the closure (Figs. 15 and 16), which is a matter of judgment. Many years ago, all wounds were left open to drain. This necessitated a second or third surgical procedure, added anesthesia, and increased hospitalization. The literature does not support adequately either decision. In 1988 a study performed at The University of Texas Southwestern Medical Center in Dallas advocated closure of amputation sites [23]. Pinzur and colleagues [24]

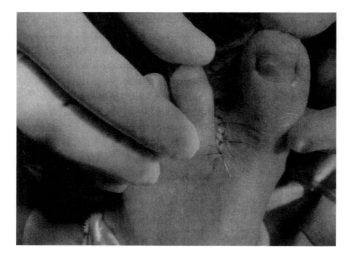

Fig. 16. Primary closure.

at Hines Veterans' Association in Illinois refuted the University of Texas study and found no difference in the outcomes of closure versus open amputations. The last study to deal with the closure of wounds was done at Wright State University School of Medicine, where a lower extemity amputation was performed on patients in sepsis and the results supported open amputation for these patients [25]. This study can be extrapolated to digital amputations, and the author believes that if a patient is septic, one should leave the amputation site open until signs of sepsis are absent and the wound edges appear viable and noninfected.

After reviewing the literature, no definitive guidelines can be formulated. The only issue that must be considered is whether all infected tissue has been resected and whether there is devitalized tissue secondary to peripheral vascular disease, which may require further wound care. The author always advises wound closure if possible, through primary means. This prevents further desiccation and devitalization of tissue and allows for a better cosmetic and functional result. In osteomyelitis and soft tissue infections of the distal phalanges, disarticulation at the proximal interphalangeal joint may be adequate, but if there is tension on the skin, the articular surface should be resected.

Surgical procedures

The most distal digital amputation is the terminal or distal Symes. It is the only named amputation of the toe. The indications for this procedure are ingrown toenails with chronic paronychia, onychomycosis, severe distal digital deformities, infections, ulcerations at the tuft of a digit, and traumatic avulsion type injuries of the distal phalanx (Fig. 17). A transverse incision over the posterior nail fold is connected to incisions on the dorsolateral and dorsomedial aspects of the phalanx. Once the incision is carried to the level of bone, resection of the distal half of the distal phalanx is performed and the plantar flap of skin is sutured

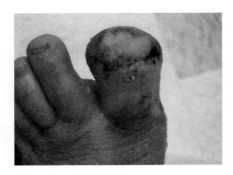

Fig. 17. Terminal Symes amputation.

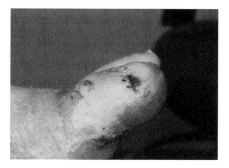

Fig. 18. Terminal Symes amputation.

to the remaining dorsal tissue (Fig. 18). Before closure, the surgeon must visualize adequate perfusion to the plantar flap and if necessary, resection of the distal phalanx at a more proximal level must be performed to ensure no tension of the skin flap. Any dog ears are resected appropriately. When performing a distal toe amputation, care should be taken to resect the entire nail bed and matrix.

The next level of amputation in the digit is at the distal interphalangeal or proximal interphalangeal joint. The approach to these joint resections may be in a dorsal to plantar or a medial to lateral orientation. The dorsal to plantar flap allows for ambulation on more durable plantar skin (Fig. 19). The medial to lateral approach to resection will allow for easier visualization of proximal tissues, but the final scar may be plantar and cause concern for future breakdown or pain (Fig. 20). Amputation of the lesser digits can be performed by resection through the phalanx or by disarticulation. If medically sound, partial digital amputation may be more beneficial than total digital amputation because a small fragment of toe will help maintain alignment of the adjacent digits. This is extremely important when dealing with a second toe amputation. If the entire

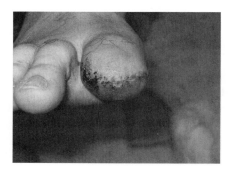

Fig. 19. Amputation with plantar to dorsal flap.

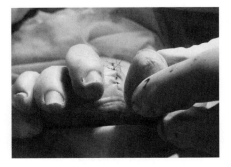

Fig. 20. Amputation with medial to lateral approach.

second digit is disarticulated at the metatarsophalangeal joint, the hallux may abduct and rotate into valgus to fill the void left by the previously amputated second digit [26].

Amputation of the hallux, similar to other digital amputations, is indicated for infection, trauma, ulcerations, and tumor. This should be performed through the proximal phalanx distal to the flexor hallucis brevis insertion. This will help maintain some stability in push-off and in the late-stance phase of gait [21,27]. Maintaining the integrity of the flexor hallucis brevis also allows for the sesamoidal apparatus to continue to function and not retract, helping to preserve plantar weight bearing and avoid transfer pressure to the second metatarsal. Seventy percent of normal toe loading is transmitted through the hallux [28]. Another normal action that may be affected post–hallux amputation is the windless effect of the plantar fascia. When this occurs, the first metatarsal bears less weight and the shift is to the lateral aspect of the foot [29]. One also may notice the development of a severe clawtoe deformity after a hallux amputation. The plantar fascia, sesamoids, and flexor hallucis brevis attach approximately 1 cm proximal to the base of the phalanx. As long as these structures are maintained, push-off can occur and allow for reduction of pressure to the lesser metatarsal heads [30].

Incisions for amputation of the great toe can be "racquet-shaped" or fish-mouth. If the racquet shape is used, carry the handle of the racquet medially at the level of the first metatarsophalangeal joint (Fig. 19). Similarly, incisions for toe amputations can be racquet or fish-mouth. The fish-mouth incisions may be closed medial to lateral or dorsal to plantar (Fig. 20). It is important not to leave dog ears and to be proximal to the disease process.

Second-digit amputations, when appropriate because of pathology, should be performed at the level of the proximal phalanx. Maintaining a stump at the base of the second toe will help prevent a hallux valgus from developing later. Disarticulation of the third or fourth digits can be performed without concern for potential deformity and the fifth digit also may be amputated without cause for concern with the gait pattern or future deformity.

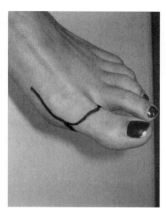

Fig. 21. Racquet incision for hallucal amputation. The more proximal the medial portion of the incision, the more of the first metatarsal can be exposed.

When faced with a decision to amputate all digits or to leave one or two digits, the author believes that a patient with one or two digits remaining may be more prone to trauma and potential complications. In this case, a transmetatarsal amputation may be a more definitive procedure with better long-term results.

Polydactyly occurs when an entire additional digit is present; polysyndactyly contains two or more bones within a single skin envelope (Fig. 21). The additional digit does not have to be functional. Poly- and syndactyly are classified by the anatomic position of the deformity. Postaxial polydactyly (fibular side) occurs about 80% of the time, preaxial (tibial side) 15% to 17% of the time, and a central duplication is seen in 3% to 6% of the cases. Polydactyly occurs in approximately one to two live births per 1000 and occurs slightly more in males. Treatment for incomplete syndactyly is not required unless a psychologic problem occurs in the child. The general surgical goal is to leave the toe with the most normal contour. More proximal osseous tissue may need to be resected with the digit, especially to decrease foot width. The timing of surgery is usu-

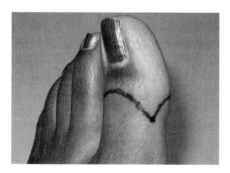

Fig. 22. Fish-mouth incision.

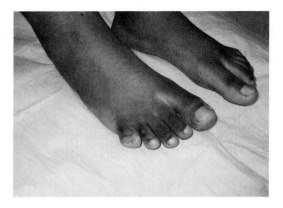

Fig. 23. Postaxial polydactyly.

ally after 1 year because of a greater potential to remodel postoperatively and for anesthetic considerations. Patients presenting at a later age generally complain of difficulty wearing conventional shoes.

Function of the foot and adjacent digits is important when selecting which digit to amputate. In the case of first or fifth digit polydactyly, usually the outermost digit is amputated. If the innermost digit demonstrates significant hypoplasia, however, it should be removed (Figs. 22–24). Central duplication is a more difficult surgical approach whereby the central digit is excised by the incision of choice. During surgery the intermetatarsal ligament must be reapproximated.

Focal gigantism of the digits or macrodactyly can be seen in isolation or in conjunction with neurofibromatosis, Klippel-Weber-Trenaunay syndrome, and Proteus syndrome [31]. Enlargement can include bone, nerve, and subcutaneous fat. Amputation of these digits will allow the patient to return to more conventional footwear and a more pleasing cosmetic appearance. Various amputations have been described.

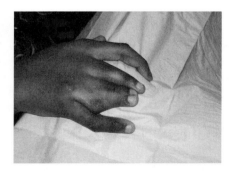

Fig. 24. The fifth finger was spared. Separation of the syndactylization resulted in the amputation of the lateralmost finger.

Box 2. ABCD guide for suspicious lesions

Asymmetry: half of the mole does not match the other half
Border: the border (edges) of the mole are ragged or irregular
Color: the color of the mole varies throughout
Diameter: the mole's diameter is larger than a pencil's eraser

Melanoma develops in cells that produce melanin (melanocytes). Melanomas cause the most deaths in skin cancers. Nevi are generally uniform in color with distinct borders. They are usually oval or round, and usually have the diameter of a pencil eraser (6 mm). The first sign of melanoma is usually a change in the existing lesion. Box 2 shows the American Academy of Dermatology's ABCD guide for suspicious lesions.

Melanomas of the nail bed or the digit will require amputation, usually at the metatarsophalangeal joint. A patient was seen with black discoloration to the distal aspect of the fifth toe. Ulceration was present to the fifth proximal interphalangeal joint and was treated as a mal perforans ulceration for 4 months. An incisional biopsy revealed a malignant melanoma (Clark's stage V, Breslow 4.0 mm) and the fifth digit was disarticulated at the metatarsophalangeal joint. The patient had a positive sentinel node. Further workup revealed metastasis to the liver, and the patient died 6 months later.

A second patient had a chronic nonhealing ingrown toenail with apparent paronychia. The patient underwent conventional treatment for same, with a partial nail avulsion and incision and drainage of the paranychia, but after 3 weeks of nonhealing the ungual labia was sent for biopsy demonstrating stage-IV, 3.4 mm melanoma. The hallux was amputated at the metatarsophalangeal joint using a racquet-shaped incision. Sentinel nodes were positive and this patient developed metastatic disease and died within 1 year.

A young adult with a pigmented lesion on the lateral aspect of the third digit distally was seen. She presented with a history of acute onset of the lesion of approximately 1 month. After excisional biopsy revealed malignant melanoma stage II, 1.2 mm, the digit was amputated at the metatarsophalangeal joint using a dorsal to plantar incision. The patient is 7 years postsurgery without recurrence of melanoma.

In these three cases, it is important to make an early diagnosis and to treat aggressively. Early treatment with stage-I and -II lesions of the digits have a good prognosis if amputation is performed either at the metatarsophalangeal joint or the transmetatarsal level.

Squamous cell carcinoma can appear similar to a cauliflower. Often these arise from small, sandpaper-like lesions called *solar* or *actinic keratoses*. They are seen more commonly in areas of sun exposure, but have been on the rise in the foot with the increased use of tanning salons. Squamous cell carcinoma also may occur in areas that have been injured previously such as burns, incisions,

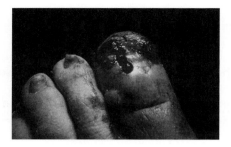

Fig. 25. Merkle-cell tumor of hallux.

and long-standing ulcers (Marjolins ulcer). Scher also has described squamous cell carcinoma of the toenail. The presentation may be as subtle as lifting of the nail plate, a verrucous-like lesion, or a recalcitrant fungal infection to a single nail plate. These should be biopsied through punch or excisonal type biopsy if small enough in diameter. If bone involvement is present, an amputation such as a distal Symes should be performed.

A 48-year-old woman with onychomycosis and a chronic verruca of the distal hallux subungually presented for care. The lesion had been present for 3 months. Initial treatment included excision of verrucoid tissue with rapid regrowth. This excised lesion was not biopsied initially because it presented as a classic appearing verruca. A punch biopsy was performed, revealing a squamous cell carcinoma with the margins extending to the periosteum of the distal phalanx. Treatment consisted of a distal Symes amputation. The patient is now 5 years postoperatively, is tumor-free, and has resumed normal activity.

Merkle cell carcinoma is a rare neoplasm of the skin. The tumor is derived from neural crest-derived Merkle cells. The tumor appears in the skin as nodules. It is highly malignant and metastasizes to the liver, bone, brain, lung, and skin. The prognosis is poor in those patients with metastatic disease. A 72-year-old woman was referred to the author with a prior diagnosis of Merkle-cell carcinoma obtained by punch biopsy of the hallux. Nodular lesions were present on the great toe of the right foot. Nodules were present for 4 months. No definitive treatment was rendered after the initial diagnosis was made. The patient underwent amputation of the great toe at the metatarsophalangeal joint through a racquet-shaped incision. The patient began chemotherapy after the amputation and 2 months later sustained a brain stem infarct and died. Postmortem revealed Merkle-cell tumor in the brain stem (Fig. 25).

Postoperative management

Postoperative healing depends directly on the patients' having adequate circulation and postoperative management, assuming that gangrenous and necrotic tissue is resected at amputation. Postoperative management should be conservative. The closed amputation should retain the sutures for 3 to 6 weeks. Strict nonweightbearing should be maintained if the patient can use crutches or a walker safely. If this is not feasible, bed rest should be ordered. Minimal complications have been identified by leaving sutures for long periods or delaying weightbearing. A broad-spectrum antibiotic generally is used in patients not allergic to penicillin. Penicillin-sensitive patients are given clindamycin routinely.

There is controversy as to whether a patient needs antibiotics if the entire infected tissue is amputated. Most agree that at least short-term postoperative antibiotics may be necessary. Sizer and Wheelock [32] stated that antibiotic coverage should be for 7 to 10 days after closed-toe amputations and 4 weeks in open amputations. The duration of antibiotics should be based on clinical findings. In many cases, if the author amputates at a level clear of infection and cellulitis, antibiotics are used for 1 week. If the wound is left open, antibiotics are used until delayed primary closure can be performed safely or at the time granulation is demonstrated with lack of clinical infection. Slow-healing wounds are an indicator of potential infection and should be recultured.

Complications

The worst complication is the failure of the primary surgical procedure. Failure may result from lack of circulation or a deterioration of distal perfusion postoperatively. It also may be related to failure to debride all necrotic tissue at the time of surgery. Lastly, failures may be attributed to additional infections away from the amputation site caused by transfer of pressure, further digital contractures, and skin tension from lack of sufficient bone resection. Hematoma within any dead space also may lead to further infection or tissue breakdown.

Complications lead to increased costs from longer or recurrent hospitalizations and can result in a more proximal amputation with loss of function and instability of the foot. Most of these complications occur when the patient has rehabilitated adequately and begins daily activity and ambulation.

Approximately 65% of hallux amputations develop a new ulceration, with 53% requiring further proximal amputation. This is in relation to lesser digital amputations in which 10% reulcerate [33]. Hammertoe deformities are common with amputation of the hallux along with metatarsalgia of the second and third metatarsophalangeal joints. As hammertoes develop, anterior displacement of the fat pad occurs and plantar problems beneath the metatarsal heads may occur. If the hammertoe is rigid, an ulcer may form dorsally over the head of the proximal phalanx. Spontaneous metatarsal fractures may be seen after digital amputation [34]. Regardless of etiology, it is important to follow all patients with amputations of the forefoot for potential transfer lesions and to treat each patient as high-risk.

Prosthetics

In the rehabilitation and prosthetic planning, it is important to keep in mind the objectives: to maintain and restore normal toe-off and propulsion, to fabricate a filler for the shoe, and to reduce transfer pressures to adjacent metatarsals and digits. Secondary concerns may include cosmesis and creating a comfortable environment in a shoe. Filling a void for digital amputations can be performed by foam fillers and by accommodative orthoses with a filler built within the device. This is not as crucial if the base of a digit is maintained.

It is of great importance to evaluate the contralateral extremity for risk factors that may lead to the demise of that foot. Many patients with amputations will undergo additional surgery, including further amputation within 5 years. Therefore accommodative devices for both feet and alternative footwear should be prescribed. Shoes with high heels increase the forefoot pressures and put the patient at further risk for injury. In many instances, extra-deep shoes with accommodative orthoses are the best means to protect the foot.

Summary

The decision to amputate a digit may be taken lightly by the surgeon, but to the patient it is extremely important. The many causes for amputation and the importance of digital amputations in the treatment of specific pathologies have been reviewed. The psychologic, mechanical, and physiologic aspects of amputations of the digits need to be considered. Good clinical judgment and adherence to sound surgical principles can make a significant difference in the results of digital amputations and in the rehabilitation of patients to normal daily function.

References

[1] Warren R, Kihn RB. A survey of lower extremity amputations for ischemia. Surgery 1968;63: 107–20.

[2] Levin M. Preventing amputation in the patient with diabetes. Diabetes Care 1995;18: 1383–91.

[3] Most R, Sinnock P. The epidemiology of lower extremity amputations in diabetic individuals. Diabetes Care 1983;6:87.

[4] Palumbo P, Melton LJ. Peripheral vascular disease and diabetes. In: Harris MI, Hamman RF, editors. Diabetes in America. NIH Publication 85–1468. Bethesda: National Institutes of Health; 1985. p. 1–21.

[5] Edmonds M, et al. Improved survival of the diabetic foot: the role of the specialized foot clinic. Q J Med 1986;232:763–71.

[6] Kominsky S. Medical and surgical management of the diabetic foot. St Louis (MO): C.V. Mosby; 1994.

[7] Wagner F. Transcutaneus doppler ultrasound in the prediction of healing and the selection of surgical level for dysvascular lesions of the toes and forefoot. Clin Orthop 1979;142:110.

[8] Goodman J, Bessman A, Teget B, et al. Risk factors in local surgical procedures for diabetic gangrene. Surg Gynecol Obstet 1976;143:587.

[9] Schwindt D, Lulloff R, Rogers S. Transmetatarsal amputations. Orthop Clin North Am 1973; 4(1):21.

[10] Bryn R. Factors influencing the healing of distal amputations performed for lower limb ischemia. Br J Surg 1992;79:73.

[11] Coldner M. The fate of the second leg in the diabetic amputee. Diabetes 1960;9:100.

[12] Crenshaw A. Campbells operative orthopedics. 7th edition. St Louis (MO): C.V. Mosby; 1987. p. 145–7.

[13] Attinger C, Venturi M, Kim K, et al. Maximizing length and optimizing biomechanics in foot amputations by avoiding cookbook recipes for amputation. Semin Vasc Surg 2003;16(1): 44–66.

[14] Holstein P. The distal blood pressure predicts healing of amputations of the feet. Acta Orthop Scand 1984;55:227.

[15] Nehler MR, Whitehill TA, Bowers SP, et al. Intermediate term outcome of primary digit amputations in patients with diabetes mellitus who have forefoot sepsis requiring hospitalization and presumed adequate circulatory status. J Vasc Surgery 1999;30(3):509–17.

[16] Rhodes GR, King TA. Delayed skin oxygenation following distal tibial revascularization (DTR): implications for wound healing in late amputations. Am Surg 1986;52:519–25.

[17] Helfet DL, Harvey T, Sanders R, et al. Limb salvage versus amputation: preliminary results of the mangled extremity severity score. Clin Orthop 1990;256:80.

[18] Gustilo RB, Anderson JT. Prevention of infection in the treatment of one thousand and twenty-five open fractures of long bones. J Bone Joint Surg Am 1976;58:453–8.

[19] Ennecking WF. Musculoskeletal tumor surgery. New York: Churchill Livingston; 1983.

[20] Carnesale PG. Benign tumors of bone. In: Crenshaw AN, editor. Campbell's operative orthopedics. 8th edition. St Louis (MO): Mosby-Yearbook; 1992. p. 235–62.

[21] Bowker JH. Partial foot amputations and disarticulations. Foot Ankle 1987;2:153.

[22] Moore JC, Jolly GP. Soft tissue considerations in partial foot amputations. Clin Podiatr Med Surg 2000;17(4):631–48.

[23] Fisher Jr DF, Clagett GP, Fry RE, et al. One-stage versus two-stage amputation for wet gangrene of the lower extremity: a randomized study. J Vasc Surg 1988;4:428–33.

[24] Pinzur MS, Smith D, Osterman H. Syme ankle disarticulation in peripheral vascular disease and diabetic infection: the one-stage versus two stage procedure. Foot Ankle Int 1995;16(3): 124–7.

[25] Scher KS, Steele FJ. The septic foot in patients with diabetes. Surgery 1988;104(4):661–6.

[26] Seligman RS, Trepal MJ, Giorgini RJ. Hallux valgus secondary to amputation of the second toe. J Am Podiatr Med Assoc 1986;76:89–91.

[27] Quill GE, Myerson MS. Clinical, radiographic and pedobarographic analysis of the foot after hallux amputation. Presented at the 58th Annual Meeting of American Academy of Orthopaedic Surgeons, Anaheim, CA, March 11, 1991.

[28] Ctercteko G, Dhanendran M, Hutton W, et al. Vertical forces acting on feet of diabetic patients with neuropathic ulcerations. Br J Surg 1981;68:608.

[29] Poppen N, Mann R, O'Konsky M, et al. Amputation of the great toe. Foot Ankle 1981;1:333.

[30] Philbin TM, Leyes M, Sferra JJ, et al. Orthopedic and prosthetic devices in partial foot amputations. Foot Ankle Clin 2001 Jun;6(2):215–28.

[31] Miura H, Uchida Y, Ihara K, et al. Macrodactyly in Proteus syndrome. J Hand Surg 1993;18B: 308–9.

[32] Sizer JS, Wheelock FC. Digital amputations in diabetic patients. Surgery 1972;72(6):980–9.

[33] Greteman B, Dale S. Digital amputations in neuropathic feet. J Am Podiatr Med Assoc 1990; 80:121.

[34] Iannucci A, et al. Spontaneous fractures of the lesser metatarsals secondary to an amputated hallux and peripheral neuropathy. J Foot Surg 1987;26:66.

ELSEVIER
SAUNDERS

Clin Podiatr Med Surg
22 (2005) 365–384

CLINICS IN
PODIATRIC
MEDICINE AND
SURGERY

Transmetatarsal Amputations

George F. Wallace, DPM, MBA*, John J. Stapleton, DPM

*Podiatry Service, University Hospital–University of Medicine and Dentistry of New Jersey,
150 Bergen Street, A-226, Newark, NJ 07103, USA*

In 1855, Bernard and Huete [1] originally described the first transmetatarsal amputation (TMA) in a patient with trench foot. In 1949, McKittrick et al [2] applied TMA for management of gangrene and diabetic foot infections. TMA originally was described as an amputation performed at the anatomic necks of the five metatarsals [2]. Today TMA is performed at various metatarsal lengths to treat a wide range of pathologies. The primary indication for TMA is the presence of a nonviable distal forefoot. The multiple causes include, but are not limited to, ulceration, failed toe and isolated ray amputations, peripheral vascular disease, trauma, embolic phenomona, frostbite, congenital deformities, and tumors. The most common indications for TMA are diabetic foot complications, peripheral vascular disease, and trauma [3]. Lawnmower injuries and motorcycle accidents are the number one reason for a traumatic TMA [3]. Performing a TMA needs to be regarded as a salvage operation for the foot and ankle surgeon and not a failure on the physician's part. TMA is used to preserve residual limb length to maintain function and reduce energy expenditure for the patient [4]. This article discusses TMAs, the decision-making process, timing of surgery, operative techniques, postoperative management, and salvage of the failed TMA.

Decision-making process

Planning begins with a detailed evaluation of the patient and the foot. The foot and ankle surgeon must take into account the ambulatory status and goals of the patient. TMA has no advantage for a bedridden patient who is nonambulatory, especially when there is any concern of healing at this distal amputation site. The

* Corresponding author.
  E-mail address: WALLACGF@UMDNJ.edu (G.F. Wallace).

more proximal amputation may be more beneficial to avoid possible surgical failure and future operations. This is especially true in patients with marked lower extremity contractures.

The overall medical status of a patient must be considered first before performing a TMA. A thorough history and physical examination should be performed on all patients. Emphasis should be placed on risk factors, such as diabetes, hypertension, peripheral vascular disease, end-stage renal disease, and smoking, that may increase the likelihood of sustaining a myocardial infarction in the perioperative period and decrease wound healing capabilities. Smoking should cease at least 1 week before surgery in nonemergent cases and throughout the postoperative course. The risk of reamputation from a complication is 2.5 times higher for smokers [5]. The patient's nutritional status and immune system must be evaluated to determine wound healing capabilities and ability to fight infection. Serum albumin and total lymphocyte count are good indicators for wound healing capabilities. Values should be greater than 3.5 g/dL and greater than $1500/mm^3$ [6]. Studies have shown that the likelihood to heal is greatly diminished when serum albumin and total lymphocyte counts are decreased [6].

Diabetic patients are often severely immunocompromised. This state can be represented as a low white blood cell count with no left shift despite the patient having an overwhelming foot infection. Fifty percent of patients with diabetes presenting with significant infection do not show typical systemic signs of fever and leukocytosis [7]. Unexplained hyperglycemia often is the only systemic indicator of infection.

Most often the need for a TMA arises emergently, and preoperative optimization is limited. The foot and ankle surgeon who is consulted for diabetic foot disorders is faced with the need to perform pedal amputations to prevent morbidity or mortality. Often after the initial skin incision it becomes evident that the infection has tracked into adjacent tissue planes, which require extensive débridement (Fig. 1). The surgeon needs to be aware that the clinical appearance of the infected diabetic foot is only the tip of the iceberg. The deep tissues usually

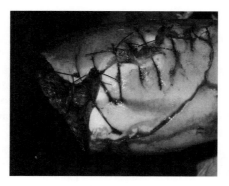

Fig. 1. TMA with delayed primary closure of a plantar incision that initially was performed to control infection tracking into the plantar central space.

are affected to a greater degree than what is visualized superficially. For this reason, with operative forefoot infections, the patient is consented and consulted on the possibility that a TMA or more proximal amputation may be needed.

Initial laboratory studies include vital signs, temperature, blood glucose, hemoglobin A_{1C}, blood cultures during fever, complete blood count with differential, complete metabolic panel, prothrombin time, activated partial thromboplastin time, international normalized ratio, sedimentation rate, C-reactive protein analysis, ECG, and x-rays. Although not often needed, the patient should be typed and crossed for a minimum of 2 U of packed red blood cells in anticipation of intraoperative bleeding.

The most important aspects of the physical examination are the factors that will determine if a TMA is indicated and the capability to heal without further complications. TMA should be performed when the first ray has been resected previously and the patient has a nonhealing ulcer under an adjacent metatarsal with or without signs of osteomyelitis. TMA also is indicated when two central rays need to be resected despite the cause. TMA should be performed for failed toe amputations that have not healed because of persistent skin breakdown and ulceration secondary to arterial insufficiency or infection (Fig. 2). The procedure also can be used for recurrent multiple neuropathic ulcerations in the absence of infection or gangrene. Although this needs to be discussed with the patient, the diabetic patient may prefer a TMA rather than having recurrent forefoot ulcerations that require multiple isolated surgical procedures, such as isolated ray resections, metatarsal head resections, and local flaps that involve increased hospitalization.

TMA is indicated for severe trauma to the distal forefoot that is unsalvageable (Fig. 3). Trauma can be the result of a motorcycle or car accident or lawnmower, industrial, gunshot, or thermal injuries. The functional outcome and ability to preserve the forefoot need to be weighed against performing a TMA. The Mangled Extremity Severity Score can be extrapolated to the foot to assist the

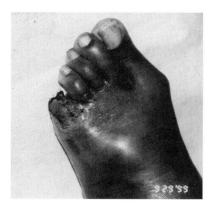

Fig. 2. Example of a failed fifth toe amputation secondary to infection that required a TMA.

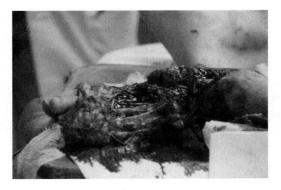

Fig. 3. Mangled extremity that required an open TMA that was revised later with skin grafts.

surgeon in deciding amputation versus limb salvage. No grading system is designated for the foot, however, to predict prognosis and treatment with regards to traumatic amputation. Clinical judgment is needed to determine the severity of the injury and to predict prognosis.

TMA can be used to treat benign and malignant tumors of the forefoot when indicated. Benign tumors may require amputation when excision compromises function and reconstruction is not feasible. TMA can be used to achieve radical resection to ensure tumor-free margins in the face of malignant tumors to the forefoot. The patient should be evaluated properly preoperatively. MRI should be performed to evaluate the extent of soft tissue or bone involvement. An incisional biopsy specimen should be obtained to establish a diagnosis and overall treatment plan. Metastatic workup should include a full-body bone scan and CT scans of the chest, abdomen, and pelvis in the face of malignant tumors. Oncology consultation should be obtained to determine the proper treatment protocol and prognosis for specific malignant tumors.

Radiographs should be obtained for all patients undergoing a TMA. In a trauma patient, the surgeon needs to evaluate the fracture pattern and degree of comminution that may exist proximal to the TMA. In the face of an acute diabetic foot infection, radiographs should be obtained quickly to determine if gas is seen in the soft tissue planes (Fig. 4). The physician should not probe ulcers before radiographs because this may cause defects in the soft tissue planes that are later difficult to distinguish from gas in the soft tissue. Ankle radiographs and proximal tibia-fibula views should be obtained if gas is seen in the foot to ensure that the level of infection has not propagated proximal into the leg. In a patient undergoing a TMA, radiographs should be evaluated to ensure that osteomyelitis is not seen proximal to the level of amputation. If there is questionable osteomyelitis, a white blood cell or HMPAO-labeled technetium bone scan or gadolinium fat-suppressed MRI should be performed to determine the presence and extent of osteomyelitis. In the presence of Charcot neuroarthropathy or in a postsurgical patient, a bone biopsy specimen should be obtained to differentiate between Charcot neuropathy and osteomyelitis.

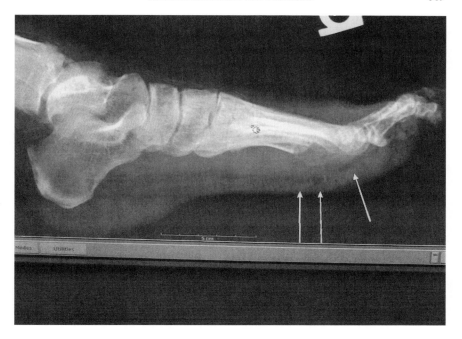

Fig. 4. Lateral radiograph of gas present in the plantar soft tissue.

The physician should evaluate vascular perfusion to the foot adequately. Initially, pulses should be palpated. A Doppler ultrasound is used if pulses are nonpalpable. Pulses that are either audible with Doppler or easily palpated in the diabetic patient have little predictive value, however, in determining the wound healing capability [8]. Noninvasive vascular studies should be ordered to determine if the amputation is likely to heal. Ankle-brachial index and pulse volume waveforms are screening tests and are not useful in a diabetic patient because they underestimate the severity of arterial insufficiency. The ankle-brachial index is affected by incompressible calcified vessels, which are common in the diabetic population and lead to falsely elevated values. Normal ankle-brachial index values and normal pulse volume waveforms in a diabetic patient have no clinical significance [9].

Transcutaneous oxygen pressure measurements ($TcPO_2$) are useful in predicting the wound healing capability at a specific level of pedal amputation [10–12]. At the authors' institution, $TcPO_2$ is the gold standard in determining the level of amputation. TMA is expected to heal if the values are greater than 30 mm Hg. One series showed a 91% healing success rate with values greater than 30 mm Hg [13]. This test can be enhanced to predict healing by administration of 100% normobaric oxygen for 20 minutes before obtaining the $TcPO_2$. It has been documented that a $TcPO_2$ value increase to 40 mm Hg or an increase of 10 mm Hg above the baseline value with administration of oxygen is predictive of successful wound healing [14–16]. Values of 20 to 30 mm Hg require a formal vascular surgical consultation for angiography and possible revascularization. Values less than 20 mm Hg indicate poor arterial perfusion that requires revascularization or transluminal angioplasty before amputation at the selected level, unless the amputation needs to be performed emergently to control infection.

In the face of acute infection that requires an emergent open TMA, vascular studies should be done postoperatively. The physician should not delay an emergent amputation because of arterial insufficiency. If revascularization is not possible, a more proximal amputation site should be chosen at a level where the $TcPO_2$ is greater than 30 mm Hg; this is easily plotted by assessing the $TcPO_2$ levels at the proposed amputation sites. Toe pressures also are used to indicate the presence of poor microcirculation to the distal forefoot. Toe pressures need to be greater than 40 mm Hg to predict successful healing at the distal forefoot [13]. If there is any question of arterial insufficiency after noninvasive vascular studies, invasive vascular studies are required to determine which lower extremity arteries are occluded, the possible collateral circulation that may be supplying distal runoff to the foot, and the mapping for future revascularization.

The skin integrity of the foot is evaluated next. The physician should estimate the amount of viable healthy skin that would remain for closure of the TMA. Often this decision cannot be made until after adequate surgical débridement of all nonviable tissue (Fig. 5). The skin flaps initially created may contract in the ensuing days postoperatively before definitive closure. It is important to look at subtle changes in the skin, such as the color, the capillary filling time, the resultant elasticity, and the thickness of the created skin flaps.

The physician needs to evaluate the foot for deformity and biomechanical disadvantages that may need to be addressed to ensure a successful TMA. Any prior ray resections that could have sacrificed the attachments of the tibialis anterior and peroneus brevis tendons require tendon transfers in conjunction with the TMA. When performing the TMA, the extensor hallucis longus and extensor digitorum longus tendons are sacrificed, and there is a loss of dorsiflexion at the

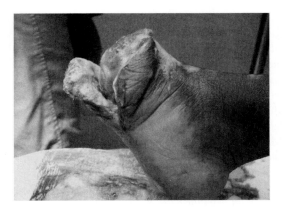

Fig. 5. Intraoperative photograph of a TMA with thick and viable skin flaps that were created after débridement and lavage.

ankle. It is imperative to evaluate the ankle joint range of motion and to determine if an equinus deformity, defined as 10° of ankle dorsiflexion with the knee flexed or extended, is present that needs to be addressed. At the authors' institution, it is protocol that an Achilles tendon lengthening or tenotomy is performed when more than half of the metatarsal shafts have been resected regardless whether equinus is present. A TMA that has a lack of dorsiflexion secondary to weak dorsiflexors or tight Achilles tendon is prone to increase pressures on the amputation site with an increased probability of future ulceration and skin breakdown.

Timing of surgery

TMA falls into two broad categories: (1) emergent cases and (2) cases that are delayed for further workup or patient optimization. Emergent TMA is indicated for diabetic foot infections, infection secondary to ischemia, or trauma. The foot and ankle surgeon faced with diabetic foot infections needs to be aware that a TMA may be a better procedure when débridement of the affected part of the foot is too extensive.

When gas is seen on radiographs or crepitation is palpated, it is imperative that the patient is brought to the operating room as soon as possible. These cases are surgical emergencies. TMAs that are performed for control of infection need to be left open to drain [17]. At the authors' institution, the sterile dressing from the initial surgery is not changed for 48 hours. At the initial dressing change, deep wound cultures are obtained. The patient may have to be premedicated with at least 2 mg of morphine sulfate intravenously if neuropathy is not present. Delayed primary closure is performed between postoperative days 3 and 5 if no vascular intervention is needed, and there are no signs of infection. There should be no growth from the deep tissue cultures, there should be a decrease in bacterial count, there should be a decrease in the white blood cell count, and the tissues should appear to be clean and viable. Only then is a revision TMA with delayed primary closure or skin graft planned.

If there is any doubt of infection or a high bacterial count of 10^5 or greater from deep quantitative cultures, the patient undergoes further débridement and pulse lavage of the wound, and the aforementioned process is repeated. If the patient requires revascularization, delayed primary closure, or skin grafting, TMA is delayed for 72 hours to ensure that a successful bypass was performed, and perfusion to the amputation site has increased. TcPO$_2$ pressure measurements can be repeated after revascularization to determine if there is a good chance that the patient will heal at the TMA level.

Additional procedures, such as tendon transfers and Achilles tendon lengthening, should be performed with closure of the TMA. Performing these ancillary procedures at this time in the presence of a clean amputation site does not lead to seeding of the infection during the initial incision, drainage, and TMA.

A patient who has sustained extensive soft tissue and bone disruption is a challenge. The Mangled Extremity Severity Score can be extrapolated to the foot to assist the surgeon in deciding on amputation versus limb salvage [18,19]. No grading system is designated for the foot, however, to predict prognosis and treatment with regard to traumatic amputation. Clinical judgment is needed to determine the severity of the injury and to predict prognosis. Mutilating injuries to the foot are surgical emergencies. The decision for emergent TMA secondary to trauma is best made in the operating room under a controlled environment after all nonviable soft tissue and bone have been removed. Major arterial injury to the limb with ischemia time of more than 6 hours requires immediate amputation [19]. The literature supports the fact that a delay in surgical intervention longer than 8 hours increases the infection rate [19–21].

At the authors' institution, severely injured patients who require a TMA are left open if the patient is brought to the operating room after 8 hours. This situation usually occurs in a patient with multiple trauma who requires precedent procedures for life-threatening injuries before foot surgery. A patient who is brought to the operating room within the golden period of 8 hours can be closed primarily at the time of surgery if all nonviable tissue and debris were removed. Severe traumatic injuries with large amounts of debris often require serial débridements before closure despite being within the golden period. The surgeon needs to determine the amount of debris and degree of contamination that was involved with the insult of injury. Lawnmower injuries are a perfect example of being inoculated with extensive debris. These injuries require serial débridements before closure. An example is type 3 open fractures according to Gustilo and Anderson [20,21].

A patient who has sustained a deep frostbite injury to the distal forefoot may require a TMA. The patient typically presents with gangrenous changes to the affected area (Fig. 6). Clinical judgment is most important to determine the timing of the TMA in this circumstance. Often with severe frostbite, demarcation of the affected area may take 3 months or longer. The TMA should be performed

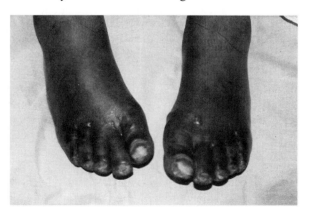

Fig. 6. Bilateral deep frostbite injury to the distal forefoot that later required TMAs.

only in the presence of infection or when the gangrene has demarcated. The proximal skin should be palpated for resilience to determine if the destructive process is still occurring. The physician should keep in mind the following aphorism when dealing with frostbite: January's frostbite is July's amputation.

Operative techniques

TMA requires detailed planning and soft tissue handling, especially in diabetic and dysvascular patients. The surgeon should use meticulous atraumatic techniques, especially with the skin. A tourniquet can be placed on the ankle or thigh per the surgeon's preference. At the authors' institution, a tourniquet is placed in case it is needed, but it is inflated only if bleeding becomes extensive. The tourniquet is contraindicated on dysvascular patients and patients who have had recent revascularization to the lower extremity. Using a tourniquet also alters the surgeon's judgment on deciding what soft tissue is viable. If a tourniquet is inflated, it should be released before closure to ensure proper hemostasis to prevent hematoma and wound dehiscence and to control bleeding.

The first step is deciding the level of amputation along the metatarsal shafts because the TMA can be performed at variable lengths. In general, one should try to preserve as much length as possible without compromising the healing process. The TMA should not be performed too far distally if there would not be adequate soft tissue coverage. When the length is determined, the incision needs to be marked out. The surgeon should mark the bases of the first and fifth metatarsals to preserve length at this region and to preserve the attachments of the tibialis anterior and peroneus brevis to improve stance and dynamic function to the residual foot.

The utilitarian incision is the fish-mouth incision, which is made with a plantar flap that is longer than the dorsal flap so that the final suture line lies on the dorsal distal aspect of the stump (Fig. 7). The contour of the flaps should be made from a distal medial–to–proximal lateral direction to avoid excessive skin after the

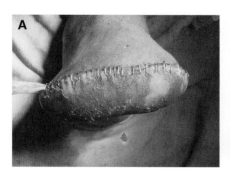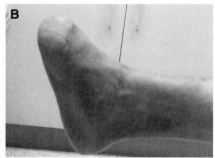

Fig. 7. (*A*) Immediate postoperative photograph of a closed TMA using a fish-mouth incision. (*B*) Postoperative photograph of a TMA.

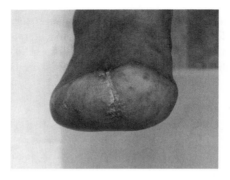

Fig. 8. Postoperative photograph of a TMA with closure of the plantar flap in a "T" fashion to excise a plantar ulcer.

bone cuts are made. This helps to prevent dog-ear formations that can be troublesome to accommodate with footwear.

The fish-mouth incision is ideal if the surgeon has a nonviolated plantar forefoot flap. An ulceration plantarly and within the forefoot flap requires the ability to create variable flap designs to provide adequate soft tissue coverage without tension to the skin. A single ulceration often can be excised in a triangular fashion and the plantar flap ultimately closed in a "T" fashion (Fig. 8).

After the initial skin incision, the incision is deepened directly down to the level of bone. There is no undermining. This incision enables the surgeon to create full-thickness flaps along the dorsal and plantar aspect of the metatarsal shafts. The dorsalis pedis artery may be transected and has to be tied off along with other bleeding vessels. Cautery is kept to a minimum if possible. At this time, the metatarsals are osteotomized completely using a sagittal saw to prevent bone regrowth and are removed with the distal forefoot. The cuts are made from dorsal distal to plantar proximal on each metatarsal with the medial and lateral aspects of the first and fifth metatarsals beveled to avoid bony prominences (Fig. 9). The metatarsal parabola needs to be maintained when making the meta-

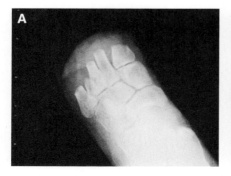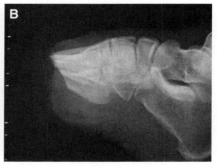

Fig. 9. (*A*) Anteroposterior radiograph of a TMA with a well-maintained metatarsal parabola. (*B*) Lateral radiograph of a TMA shows the angulation of the bone cuts to avoid a plantar prominence.

tarsal bone cuts. Attention is directed to removing all tendons within the flaps that were created. Traction should be placed on the flexor and extensor tendons with a Kocher and transected as far proximally as possible. It is imperative to remove the plantar plates and the sesamoids because these structures can become prominent against the plantar flap.

Proper débridement is essential in the face of infection. The surgeon needs to figure out where the infection is tracking to remove all infected tissue adequately. The tendon sheaths need to be inspected for purulence. At times, the surgeon has to extend the initial incision or place another skin incision to ensure the infection is not tracking further proximal or into the leg (Fig. 10). After all nonviable tissue has been removed, the wound should be pulse lavaged with at least 3 L of normal saline in addition to 3 L of normal saline mixed with polymyxin and bacitracin. There has been debate that the pulse lavage can seed superficial bacteria deep into the wound because of the high pressures that are created [22]. Surgeons can use a Versajet (Smith & Nephew Wound Management, Largo, Florida), which can remove debris and débride tissue via a high-velocity water jet that can be controlled. The Versajet also can débride tissue superficially with fine control, which may limit the amount of tissue that would have to be removed.

After proper irrigation and débridement, the operating team should change the outer pair of gloves to avoid contamination; a wound culture is obtained, which determines if the initial débridement was adequate. Unused instrumentation is used from this point on. Drapes also should be changed. The infected TMA or the traumatic amputation that was performed outside the golden period needs to be packed open and local wound care continued until there are no signs of infection before any closure. The wound can be packed with iodoform 0.5-inch packing soaked in saline, then dressed with a dry sterile dressing.

Proper repeat débridement also needs to be performed on revision TMAs before closure; this occurs minimally 3 days after the initial surgery. It is imperative to excise the wound margins sharply to create an acute wound, curet granulation tissue, freshen the bone margins and pulse lavage the wound before

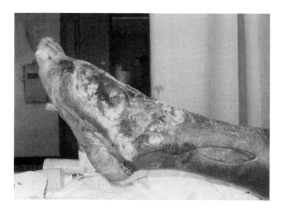

Fig. 10. Example of an infection that tracked proximal into the leg.

delayed primary closure. Closure of the TMA should be performed with minimal skin tension to prevent necrosis. The skin should be approximated, and any redundancy should be sharply excised. If tension is apparent, further bone resection or slight thinning of the flap may be necessary. The subcutaneous tissues are coapted and sutured with a few simple absorbable sutures. The skin is approximated and either stapled or sutured using a low reactive suture, such as polypropylene. The skin should be sutured in the middle and at the medial and lateral edges first with subsequent sutures bisecting the adjacent sutures until the wound is closed. Suturing in this manner prevents the formation of dog ears at the medial and lateral aspects. A drain can be used as needed.

Patients who were found to have an equinus deformity on initial examination or proximal TMA require an Achilles tendon lengthening or tenotomy during closure of the TMA. A proximal TMA is defined as half or more of the metatarsals being transected (Fig. 11). A longitudinal open procedure and percutaneous approach have been described in the literature [23]. At the authors' institution, a percutaneous triple hemisection Achilles tendon lengthening is performed on all nondiabetic patients who require an Achilles tendon lengthening. In diabetic patients, the authors perform a percutaneous snap tenotomy through a medial stab incision located 1.5 to 2 cm from the insertion of the Achilles tendon. The tenotomy is performed as opposed to the lengthening to prevent recurrence of the equinus deformity. Diabetic patients with a hyperglycemic state are prone to nonenzymatic glycosylation of the Achilles tendon, which results in a loss of elasticity and recurrence of the equinus deformity.

Patients who require a TMA with a nonviable plantar flap, whether secondary to infection, trauma, or thermal injuries, may require a guillotine TMA with future skin grafting, synthetic grafting, or closure by secondary intention (Fig. 12). The guillotine TMA should be performed initially and packed open with wet-to-dry dressings. The physician should inspect the wound in 48 hours to determine if there is an adequate amount of granulation tissue. The wound also should be assessed for signs of infection. Deep tissue should be obtained for culture and for

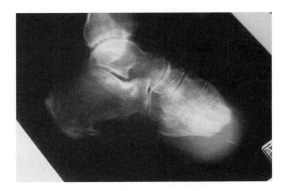

Fig. 11. Lateral radiograph of a proximal TMA that required an Achilles tenotomy by definition of more than half of the metatarsal shafts being transected.

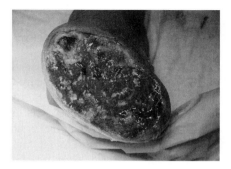

Fig. 12. Guillotine TMA performed secondary to infection.

quantitative bacterial counts before skin grafting. Grafts, whether skin or synthetic, require a healthy granular base (Fig. 13). A vacuum-assisted closure device can be used to accelerate granulation tissue before skin grafting. With meticulous wound care, the physician can promote abundant granulation tissue that can epithelialize by secondary intention [17,24].

In wounds that are to be grafted, the borders of the wound should be sharply excised with a minimal amount of soft tissue loss to promote neoepithialization with onlay of a split-thickness skin graft (STSG). Before onlay of the STSG, the granular bed is débrided again with a curet and pulse lavaged with 3 L of normal saline followed by 3 L of normal saline mixed with polymyxin and bacitracin. A Versajet also can be used at this stage to create an optimal bed before skin grafting.

At the authors' institution, meshed STSGs harvested from the ipsilateral lateral calf typically are used. The thickness of the STSG typically is harvested at 18/1000 inch. At this thickness, there is the greatest likelihood of graft take, while minimizing the amount of skin graft contracture. Before applying the skin graft, adequate hemostasis is achieved. Then the STSG is applied and trimmed as needed and secured using either staples or simple polypropylene sutures. Cotton soaked in mineral oil is applied over the STSG with fluffs and a dry sterile

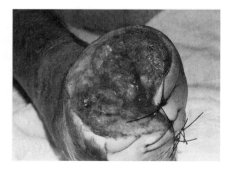

Fig. 13. Guillotine TMA after vacuum-assisted closure to create a healthy granular base for skin grafting.

compressive stent dressing. A posterior splint is applied to the lower extremity. The patient can be discharged the next day. The first dressing change after this skin graft typically is 5 to 7 days postoperatively.

In a trauma patient who requires a TMA, the same operative techniques apply with the exception that at times antecedent trauma, in the form of open or closed fractures, neurovascular insult, or soft tissue injuries, has to be addressed in conjunction with performing a TMA. It is often necessary to stabilize fractures in the residual foot with either Kirschner wires or external fixation. External fixation often is chosen because it allows the surgeon the opportunity to stabilize fractures, correct any angular deformities, maintain length, immobilize the affected foot and ankle, and allow wound care as required. Internal fixation should not be used in contaminated or infected wounds. External fixation also is applicable to closed or limited open surgical techniques. External fixation is an excellent modality to sustain length to severely comminuted or absent bone fragments that will require later bone grafting.

Trauma patients who present with acute vascular compromise to either the dorsalis pedis or the posterior tibial artery need to be handled efficiently. Initially in the emergency department, a pneumatic ankle tourniquet should be placed on the ankle. Before inflation, the physician needs to access the source of the bleeding. If the dorsalis pedis artery is affected, the artery should be tied off in the emergency department if possible. If hemostasis cannot be achieved, the pneumatic ankle tourniquet should be inflated and the patient brought to the operating room emergently to ligate the dorsalis pedis within a controlled environment. The dorsalis pedis supplies approximately 15% of the blood flow to the foot, so repair of the vessel is not necessary. The posterior tibial artery supplies most of the blood flow to the foot. If the posterior tibial artery was severed, the pneumatic ankle tourniquet should be placed and inflated initially in the emergency department and the patient brought emergently to the operating room for repair of the artery.

Various types of soft tissue injury to the residual lower extremity can be associated with a traumatic TMA. Often the residual foot or leg has sustained severe crush, degloving, thermal, and mutilating injuries. Myerson's split-thickness skin excision [3] can be useful in determining tissue viability and zone of injury in crush and degloving injuries. The technique involves harvesting an STSG from the injured and uninjured skin. When the STSG is harvested, the zone of viability is determined by the presence of dermal capillary bleeding. Nonviable areas are excised and grafted with the meshed STSG that was harvested earlier. Fluorescein labeling also can be used to determine tissue viability. Fluorescein, in a dose of 10 mg/kg intravenously, fluoresces under UV light in the presence of viable skin that has an intact capillary bed [3]. Wounds that are embedded with large amounts of debris require meticulous débridements with pulsatile lavage that are repeated until a clean wound is obtained.

Various types of benign and malignant tumors of the foot can be treated with a TMA when indicated. A TMA should be performed to achieve wide or radical resection of malignant tumors. A TMA can be performed to excise extensive benign tumors to enhance function.

Postoperative management

Postoperative management is crucial in preventing failure of the TMA. The most important part is patient compliance. The physician-patient relationship is crucial at this time to prevent future problems.

Initially after surgery, the foot is elevated (with the exception of vascular patients) to prevent edema. Edema control is important in the postoperative period. Often with poor edema control, verrucous hyperplasia is seen that can lead to future skin breakdown. The physician must prevent ulceration to the residual foot, so the foot should be offloaded to prevent pressure to the heel. In an open TMA, the sterile dressing should be kept intact for 48 hours before the first dressing change as described previously. Partial weight bearing with heel touch in a surgical shoe is allowed. The closed TMA can be placed in a surgical shoe and partial weight bearing allowed. Patients with delicate skin and poor soft tissue coverage should be non–weight bearing until the skin incision has healed and the sutures are removed. Physical therapy should be used so that the patient can comply with the weight-bearing restrictions and to fit the patient properly with the appropriate gait assistive devices.

The surgical dressing on the closed TMA should be changed 3 to 5 days postoperatively. The TMA that required skin grafting should be placed in a posterior splint to eliminate motion if an external fixation device was not used. The compressive dressing over the STSG should not be changed for 5 to 7 days. At the authors' institution, it has not been necessary to keep a patient with an STSG bedridden and hospitalized with strict elevation for the initial 5 to 7 days. If a patient had an Achilles tenotomy in conjunction with a TMA, there is no change in the dressing or weight-bearing status. Patients who had a percutaneous Achilles tendon lengthening in conjunction with a TMA are placed in a posterior splint in slight dorsiflexion and are instructed to be non–weight bearing for 6 to 8 weeks.

After closure of the TMA, the patient should be seen weekly. The time for suture or staple removal is generally around 3 weeks postoperatively. Diabetic patients may require additional time if there are any signs of delayed healing. The incision should be inspected to ensure it is well coapted without dehiscence or signs of infection. An open TMA that is healing by secondary intention should be treated with local wound care. Roach et al [24] reported successful healing at an average of 2 months, with open midfoot amputations that healed by secondary intention. STSGs when used should be evaluated for signs of hematoma, seroma, and infection that could lead to graft failure.

The physician ideally should see the patient weekly for the first month, then every 2 weeks for the next 2 months if there are no complications with the TMA. The literature states that wound complications or skin breakdown at a TMA site typically occurs within 3 months postoperatively [25]; however, this does not imply that the patient is not closely followed after 3 months.

The most common complications encountered during the rehabilitative course are skin breakdown and a feeling of instability during normal activities [26].

These complications can be reduced greatly with custom-molded shoes. Patients who are fitted with custom-made shoes and insoles have been shown to have decreased plantar pressures compared with patients who have regular shoes with toe fillers [27]. The use of a rigid rocker-bottom sole or carbon fiber plate can assist significantly in physical performance with increased walking speeds [27,28]. Ankle-foot orthoses generally restrict ankle joint range of motion and can become cumbersome to fit properly with shoe gear. Patients must be counseled on the importance of wearing only professionally designed shoes. In diabetic patients, it has been shown that plantar forefoot pressures after a TMA are increased [29]. Through proper footwear, the weight can be distributed properly to decrease these peak plantar pressures [27].

In diabetic and vascular patients, a preventive care program is established. The diabetic patient should be taught to inspect the feet regularly, especially at the amputation site, for any signs of skin breakdown or infection. Patients should have regular follow-up appointments with their primary physician, podiatric surgeon, endocrinologist, vascular surgeon, and pedorthotist. Blood glucose values should be well controlled by the primary care physician or endocrinologist with hemoglobin A_{1C} levels less than 7. Patients also should be made aware and understand the importance of their hemoglobin A_{1C} level. Patients should have serial vascular examinations to prevent limb loss secondary to ischemia. Smokers should be involved in a smoking cessation program to eliminate a major risk factor in the development of peripheral vascular disease and future amputations. The postoperative management of the amputee is an ongoing process of observation and early intervention when needed. The contralateral limb is routinely inspected at the same time as the TMA site.

Revision transmetatarsal amputation

TMA can be an excellent amputation stump to provide the patient with good function and less energy expenditure than more proximal amputations [4]. TMA is associated with higher revision rates, however, compared with more proximal amputations, such as the below-knee and above-knee amputation [30,31]. Revision TMAs are higher in diabetic and vascular patients with rates of 30% to 40% [30,31]. Reamputation rates are higher among women and the elderly [32]. Lower temperature at the amputation site also is a risk factor for reampuation [32].

Reducing the need for a revision TMA begins with the proper preoperative evaluation and selecting an appropriate amputation level, operative techniques, and postoperative management. Even with the most meticulous planning and operative techniques, the surgeon is faced at times with revision TMA, especially in a neuropathic patient who is prone to skin breakdown. Revision surgery at the TMA level is indicated for, but not limited to, skin breakdown, soft tissue and bone infection, necrosis, bony prominences, stump neuroma, and deformity.

Reevaluation of the postamputation patient is necessary to determine the cause of skin breakdown, pain, or instability.

Skin breakdown can be caused by numerous factors. The presence of infection can be the underlying cause, especially in a diabetic patient with a limited host defense mechanism. Often the first signs of underlying osteomyelitis are ulcers without clinical signs of infection. Physical examination, white blood cell count, sedimentation rate, C-reactive protein analysis, and radiographs are the initial evaluation tests to determine the presence of osteomyelitis or deep soft tissue infection. White blood cell scans are helpful to determine the presence of osteomyelitis when radiographs are equivocal. CT and MRI can help define the extent of osteomyelitis. When osteomyelitis is determined, bone resection should be planned. A dilemma develops: Should a more proximal TMA be undertaken, or is it more prudent to perform a more proximal (Lisfranc, Chopart, Symes, or below-knee) amputation? Antibiotic beads can be placed to achieve a high local concentration of antibiotics while closing the wound primarily. The physician also should be aware of the possibility of methicillin-resistant *Staphylococcus aureus* when patients continue to have recurrent skin breakdown after receiving several courses of antibiotics. Linezolid serves as an excellent treatment option for this specific patient population.

Bony prominences in the form of prominent bone cuts, osseous regrowth, or musculoskeletal deformity can directly cause skin breakdowns (Fig. 14). Radiographs and CT scans should be evaluated closely to delineate bony prominences. Bony prominences should be removed surgically to avoid future breakdown. It is imperative to make bone cuts with a powered saw to avoid bone regrowth. The literature supports the fact that bone regrowth can be prevented by the burning of bone that occurs with the use of a powered saw and when bone cuts are performed away from the metaphysis of the bone. Male gender also is a risk

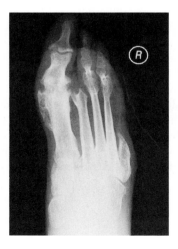

Fig. 14. Anteroposterior radiograph shows bony regrowth.

factor for bone regrowth [33]. The foot should be examined for a residual or recurrent equinus deformity with distal ulcerations or skin breakdown. An Achilles tendon lengthening or tenotomy should be performed if not done already. At times, the posterior ankle joint capsule needs to be released to achieve dorsiflexion. If an equinus deformity persists despite addressing the soft tissue contractures, an arthrodesis procedure to correct the deformity may have to be considered. Ankle arthrodesis in slight dorsiflexion for a TMA patient with adequate vascular supply is an excellent alternative procedure to prevent future ulceration and proximal amputation secondary to skin breakdown from the equinus deformity.

In a vascular patient, failed TMA is usually the result of poor selection of amputation level or when the revascularization fails or clogs at a time far removed from the initial procedure [34]. TcPO$_2$ can indicate the probability of wound healing. Vascular surgical intervention is often the only way to salvage a failed TMA secondary to peripheral vascular disease [34]. After revascularization, the possibility of further resection cannot be ruled out. A more proximal amputation is often the only way to salvage a failed TMA if revascularization is not possible.

In a trauma patient, wound complications and skin breakdown are usually the result of poor tissue coverage. The surgeon may have used thin traumatized skin to cover the amputation site or applied STSGs on weight-bearing areas or over bony prominences. Wounds of limited depth and size are amenable to local wound care, local tissue flaps, and STSGs if a healthy granular bed can be obtained. The surgeon has to become creative in using tissue and remodeling the bony architecture at times to obtain closure of a failed TMA.

For larger defects with adequate vascular supply, microsurgical free muscle flaps are an excellent alternative to salvage a failed TMA. The surgical management of a failed TMA requires early recognition and appreciation of underlying disease characteristics that may compromise a successful amputation.

Summary

TMA is an excellent procedure in the face of nonhealing ulceration, infection, trauma, peripheral vascular disease, and tumors. Proper decision planning, timing of surgery, operative techniques, and postoperative management are fundamental to the reduction of failures associated with TMA. Even with awareness and knowledge, unforeseen failures are inevitable. The physician needs to accept this notion and establish the underlying cause for failure to revise a TMA properly.

References

[1] Bernard C, Huete C, quoted in Schwindt CD, Lulloff RS, Rogers SC. Transmetatarsal amputations. Orthop Clin North Am 1973;4:31–42.

[2] McKittrick LS, McKittrick JB, Risley TS. Transmetatarsal amputation for infection or gangrene in patients with diabetes mellitus. Ann Surg 1949;130:826–42.

[3] Myerson M. Management of crush injuries and compartment syndromes of the foot. In: Myerson M, editor. Foot and ankle disorders. Philadelphia: WB Saunders; 2003. p. 1229–31.

[4] Waters RL, Perry J, Antonelli D, Hislop H. Energy cost of walking of amputees: the influence of length of amputation. J Bone Joint Surg 1976;58A:42–51.

[5] Lind J, Kramhoff M, Bodker S. The influence of smoking on complications after primary amputations of the lower extremity. Clin Orthop 1991;267:211–7.

[6] Pinzur M, Kaminisky M, Sage R, Cronin R, Osterman H. Amputations at the middle level of the foot. J Bone Joint Surg 1986;68A:1061.

[7] Encroth M, Apelquist J, Stenstrom A. Clinical characteristics and outcome in 223 diabetic patients with deep foot infections. Foot Ankle Int 1997;18:716–22.

[8] Welch GH, Leiberman DP, Pollock JG, Angerson W. Failure of Doppler ankle pressure to predict healing of conservative forefoot amputations. Br J Surg 1985;72:888–9.

[9] Goss DE, de Trafford J, Roberts VC, Flynn MD, Edmonds ME, Watkins PJ. Raised ankle/brachial pressure index in insulin-treated diabetic patients. Diabet Med 1989;6:576–8.

[10] Ballard JL, Eke CC, Bunt TJ, Killeen JD. A prospective evaluation of transcutaneous oxygen measurements in the management of diabetic foot problems. J Vasc Surg 1995;22:485.

[11] Bunt TJ, Hollway GA. TcPo$_2$ as an accurate predictor of therapy in limb salvage. Ann Vasc Surg 1996;10:224.

[12] Misuri A, Lucertini G, Nanni A, Viacava A, Belardi P. Predictive value of transcutaneous oximetry for selection of amputation level. J Cardiovasc Surg (Torino) 2000;41:83–7.

[13] Bowers BL, Valentine RJ, Myers SI, Chervu A, Clagett GP. The natural history of patients with claudication with toe pressures of 40 mm Hg or less. J Vasc Surg 1993;18:506–11.

[14] Harward TR, Volny J, Golbranson F, Bernstein EF, Fronek A. Oxygen inhalation-induced transcutaneous Po$_2$ changes as a predictor of amputation level. J Vasc Surg 1993;18:506–11.

[15] McCollum PT, Spence VA, Walker WF. Oxygen induced changes in the skin as measured by transcutaneous oximetry. Br J Surg 1986;73:882.

[16] Sheffield PJ. Tissue oxygen measurements. In: Davis JC, Hunt TK, editors. Problem wounds: the role of oxygen. New York: Elseiver; 1988. p. 17.

[17] Durham JR, McCoy DM, Sawchuk AP, et al. Open transmetatarsal amputation in the treatment of severe foot infections. Am J Surg 1989;158:127–30.

[18] Helfet DL, Howey T, Sanders R, Johansen K. Limb salvage versus amputation: preliminary results of the mangled extremity severity score. Clin Orthop 1990;256:80.

[19] Johansen K, Daines M, Howey T, et al. Objective criteria accurately predict amputation following lower extremity trauma. J Trauma 1990;30:568.

[20] Gustillo RB, Anderson JJ. Prevention of infection in the treatment of one thousand and twenty five open fractures of long bones: retrospective and prospective analysis. J Bone Joint Surg Am 1976;58:453–8.

[21] Gustillo B, Merlcow RL, Templemen D. The management of open fractures. J Bone Joint Surg Am 1990;72:299–303.

[22] Peregudou IG, Zubarev PN, Isupou I. Pulse jet administration of liquid in the treatment of suppurative wounds. Vestn Khir Im I I Grek 1989;142:58–60.

[23] Hatt RN, Lamphier TA. Triple hemisection: a simplified procedure for lengthening the achilles tendon. N Engl J Med 1947;236:166–9.

[24] Roach JJ, Deutsch A, McFarlane DS. Resurrection of the amputations of LisFranc and Chopart for diabetic gangrene. Arch Surg 1987;122:931.

[25] Mueller MJ, Allen BT, Sinacore DR. Incidence of skin breakdown and higher amputation after transmetatarsal amputation: implications for rehabilitation. Arch Phys Med Rehabil 1995; 76:50–4.

[26] Mueller MJ, Sinacore DR. Rehabilitation factors following transmetatarsal amputation. Phys Ther 1994;74:1027–33.

[27] Mueller MJ, Strube MJ, Allen BT. Therapeutic footwear can reduce plantar pressures in patients with diabetes and transmetatarsal amputation. Diabetes Care 1997;20:637–41.

[28] Tang SF, Chen CP, Chen MJ, Chen WP, Leong CP, Chu NK. Transmetatarsal amputation prosthesis with carbon fiber plate: enhanced gait function. Am J Phys Med Rehabil 2004; 83:123–30.

[29] Garbalosa JC, Cavanagh PR, Wu G, et al. Foot function in diabetic patients after partial amputation. Foot Ankle 1996;17:43.

[30] Hosch J, Quiroga C, Bosma J, Peters EJ, Armstrong DG, Lavery LA. Outcomes of transmetatarsal amputations with diabetes mellitus. J Foot Ankle Surg 1997;36:430–4.

[31] Larsson V, Anderson G. Partial amputation of the foot for diabetic or arteriosclerotic gangrene. J Bone Joint Surg 1978;60B:126–30.

[32] Ohsawa S, Inamori Y, Fukuda K, Hirotuji M. Lower limb amputation for diabetic foot. Arch Orthop Trauma Surg 2001;121:186–90.

[33] Armstrong DG, Hadi S, Nguyen HC, Harkless LB. Factors associated with bone regrowth following diabetes related partial amputations of the foot. J Bone Joint Surg 1999;11:1561–5.

[34] Glass H, Rowe VL, Houd DB. Influence of transmetatarsal amputation in patients requiring lower extremity distal revascularization. Am Surg 2004;70:845–9.

ELSEVIER
SAUNDERS

Clin Podiatr Med Surg
22 (2005) 385–393

CLINICS IN
PODIATRIC
MEDICINE AND
SURGERY

Lisfranc and Chopart Amputations

Mark A. DeCotiis, DPM[a,b,c,*]

[a]*Podiatry Service, University Hospital–UMDNJ, 150 Bergen Street, A-226, Newark, NJ 07103, USA*
[b]*Curative Wound Care Center, Bayshore Community Hospital, 727 North Beers Street,
Holmdel, NJ 07733, USA*
[c]*Private Practice, 721 North Beers Street, Holmdel, NJ 07733, USA*

The issue of choosing an amputation level can be difficult for physicians. Every attempt should be made to maintain as much pedal length as possible to increase biomechanical function and ambulatory power. The transmetatarsal amputation is probably the most common amputation performed today. When there is excessive soft tissue loss because of trauma, infection, or vascular compromise, however, a Lisfranc amputation should be considered as another limb-salvage procedure.

History

Jacques Lisfranc de St. Martin was a French gynecologist and surgeon. He obtained his medical degree in 1813 when he served as an assistant to Guillamme Depuytren. In addition to multiple gynecologic procedures, Lisfranc devised a technique to treat forefoot gangrene by partial amputation of the foot. Not only does the amputation bear his name, but also the tarsometatatarsal joint is referred to as *Lisfranc's joint*. Lisfranc was well known for his ability to amputate a foot in less than 1 minute [1].

Indications

The primary indication for a Lisfranc amputation is extensive soft tissue loss of the forefoot, which prevents a successful transmetatarsal amputation. The cause of this soft tissue loss can be attributed to many different factors, includ-

---

* Curative Wound Care Center, Bayshore Hospital, 727 North Beers Street, Holmdel, NJ 07733.
E-mail address: drmadecotiis@msn.com

0891-8422/05/$ – see front matter © 2005 Elsevier Inc. All rights reserved.
doi:10.1016/j.cpm.2005.03.012   *podiatric.theclinics.com*

ing diabetes, peripheral vascular disease, osteomyelitis, soft tissue infection, and trauma. The primary goal of any pedal amputation is to maintain as much fore-foot length as possible to improve biomechanical function. A Lisfranc amputation is not indicated for a nonambulatory patient; in these cases, a more proximal amputation should be considered. When distal procedures have failed, and one has adequate soft tissue viability to perform a Lisfranc amputation, this amputation level is a viable option to preserve length of the foot, allowing patients to be functional in a modified shoe rather than a prosthesis.

General considerations

Many factors should be considered when determining an amputation level. The most important determinant of healing potential is vascular supply. The choice of an amputation must be at a level where there is adequate perfusion to the tissues [2]. A thorough preoperative vascular workup should be performed before any pedal amputation. This workup should include arterial Doppler studies and transcutaneous oxygen measurements to gauge tissue perfusion and viability [3]. When necessary, a vascular consultation should be obtained to determine if lower extremity revascularization is indicated before performing any amputation to increase healing potential. This full vascular workup also may prevent unnecessary surgery in a patient who does not have adequate perfusion to heal.

The patient's overall health and nutritional status also should be evaluated. Medical and endocrinology consultations should be obtained before surgery to maintain strict control of glucose levels during the perioperative period. This control optimizes the patient's ability to heal and fight infection.

When the decision is made to perform a Lisfranc amputation, one should consider the musculotendinous structures that are going to be encountered during this procedure, including the tibialis posterior, peroneal, and tibialis anterior tendons. The tibialis posterior tendon has its main insertion to the base of the navicular, then extends to the bases of the second and third metatarsals and the cuneiforms. The action of this muscle is to provide inversion and plantar flexion of the foot. The insertion should be preserved because its main navicular insertion is not encountered during the procedure. The attachments to the plantar aspect of the cuneiforms should be preserved as much as possible, however.

The peroneus brevis and tertius insert into the base of the fifth metatarsal and the cuboid. These muscles are powerful evertors of the foot, and their insertions should be preserved if possible. It is the author's preference to maintain the base of the fifth metatarsal during this procedure to maintain full power of the peroneus brevis; however, if this is not feasible, leaving as much of the insertion as possible is important to maintain function. If necessary, this tendon can be reattached to the cuboid or sutured to the surrounding soft tissue. The tibialis anterior tendon has its insertion into the base of the first metatarsal and medial cuneiform. It is a powerful dorsiflexor of the foot. Its attachment should be preserved when possible and if disturbed should be reattached to the proximal aspect of the medial cuneiform to preserve function.

These musculotendinous structures are important to maintain positioning and function of the foot. Keeping as much of the insertions of these muscles intact and performing tendon transfers when able to do so are essential to create a functional amputation and to avoid future complications.

Because of the proximity of this amputation, and the loss of function of the muscles described previously, the Achilles tendon gains a mechanical advantage, and a residual equinovarus deformity can occur. To avoid this complication, an Achilles tendon lengthening or complete tenotomy should be performed. In the presence of an infection, any Achilles tendon procedure should be performed at a later date, when the patient's wound is free of infection. It is the author's preference to perform a complete tenotomy of the Achilles tendon routinely because more than half the length of the foot is lost during a Lisfranc amputation. In addition, many of the dorsiflexors of the foot have been disrupted, and the posterior tibial tendon should create sufficient plantar flexion during gait. An Achilles tendon tenotomy or lengthening should be performed in addition to, and not in place of, adequate musculotendinous balancing procedures.

Surgical technique

Meticulous handling of the soft tissues, especially for patients with diabetes or vascular compromise, is paramount when performing any foot amputation. Special attention should be paid to maintaining as much soft tissue as possible to allow for adequate closure under minimal tension. Preoperatively, it may be helpful to design the flaps with a skin marker. A fish-mouth flap should be designed as illustrated in Fig. 1. The dorsal flap should be made slightly distal

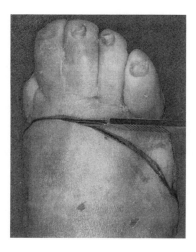

Fig. 1. Dorsal incision for Lisfranc amputation.

to the amputation level, and the plantar flap should be fashioned longer to allow for closure.

Full-thickness flaps should be maintained dorsally and plantarly. During the dorsal dissection, special care should be taken to locate and ligate the dorsalis pedis artery. When a full-thickness flap is created, a periosteal elevator is used to elevate the soft tissue overlying the tarsometatarsal articulation plantarly and dorsally. Special care should be taken to preserve the muscles described previously during the dissection. When necessary, these tendons should be transferred to proximal structures. The long flexor and extensor tendons should be clamped, pulled distally, and transected. These tendons also should be inspected for the presence of infection tracking proximally into the rear foot or leg.

Disarticulation of the metatarsals is now performed. Meticulous handling and retraction of the tissues is vital during the disarticulation process. During the disarticulation, the bases of the second and fifth meatatarsals should be salvaged to maintain their muscular attachments. In addition, the base of the second metatarsal is recessed proximally, and by leaving the base a good parabola is created. When the disarticulation is complete, any bony prominences or potential source of ulceration should be rongeured or rasped smooth. The wound should be irrigated copiously using a pulsed lavage system before closure. It may be necessary because of infection to leave the amputation site open and return to the operating room for delayed closure.

Before closure of the plantar flap, it should be debulked to allow for adequate closure under minimal tension. This debulking process can be performed with a no. 10 scalpel blade or Metzenbaum scissors. Special care should be taken not to remove excessive tissue from the plantar flap, dysvascularizing the flap. The dorsal and plantar flaps are reapproximated to assess ease of closure (Fig. 2).

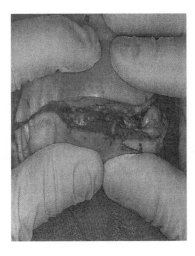

Fig. 2. Reapproximation of wound after disarticulation.

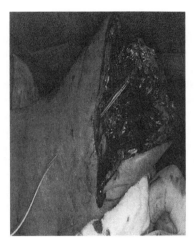

Fig. 3. Drain in place.

Before closure, a closed suction drain is preferable to prevent hematoma formation (Fig. 3). Closure is performed using 3-0 absorbable sutures placed through the deep fascia. Skin is reapproximated using 3-0 monofilament suture in a horizontal-type fashion to allow for eversion of skin edges. Large bites of tissue on both sides of the incision line are necessary to prevent the sutures from pulling through secondary to postoperative swelling. The incision site should be dressed with an antibiotic-impregnated gauze and a well-padded bandage to prevent trauma to the amputation site postoperatively (Fig. 4).

Postoperative care

The patient is placed in a well-padded posterior splint postoperatively to protect the amputation site and provide immobilization for a concomitant Achilles tendon procedure. If a closed suction drain is used, it should be

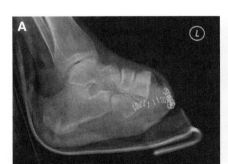
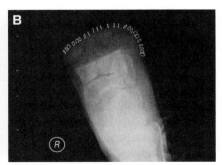

Fig. 4. (*A* and *B*) Radiographs after amputation.

discontinued within 24 to 48 hours depending on the amount of drainage. When drainage is less than 10 to 20 mL during a 24-hour period, the drain should be removed. If drainage occurs in excess of this amount for an extended period, one should be concerned about active bleeding and should return to the operating room to achieve hemostasis if necessary. The patient is kept non–weight bearing for at least 3 weeks until the incision is healed. If an Achilles tendon lengthening is performed, immobilization should be continued a minimum of 6 weeks. The timing of suture removal is a clinical decision. With an amputation of this type, the author prefers to leave sutures in a minimum of 3 weeks. When the patient is ready to ambulate, he or she should be professionally fitted in a custom-molded shoe with a filler to accommodate the amputated forefoot. The patient should be instructed to examine the amputation site daily and should be monitored closely for any complications to the amputation site and the contralateral limb resulting from excessive pressure.

Complications

Complications of the Lisfranc amputation are similar to complications of the transmetatarsal amputation and include necrosis of the incision line, equinovarus deformity, delayed healing, and postoperative infection. Each of these complications is discussed with suggestions on how to avoid them.

Necrosis of the incision line

Most pedal amputations are performed on patients with diabetes or vascular compromise or both. Meticulous, gentle handling of the soft tissues is essential to healing. In addition, closing the amputation under minimal tension is important; special care should be taken in debulking the plantar flap and resecting adequate bone to allow for easy closure.

Equinovarus deformity

As a result of the loss of most of the dorsiflexors and the shortening of the foot, the Achilles tendon gains increased power, leading to equinovarus deformity. Ulceration of the distal stump can be a direct result of equinovarus deformity. Salvaging muscular attachments when possible and performing appropriate musculotendinous balancing procedures and an Achilles tendon tenotomy are imperative in creating a functional amputation and avoiding an equinovarus deformity.

Delayed healing

Delayed healing is most likely a function of the patient population that requires a pedal amputation. Most amputations today are performed on suboptimal patients. Controlling infection during the perioperative period, optimizing the patient's medical and nutritional status, and performing a full preoperative vascular assessment can minimize complications. It is also important to counsel patients preoperatively so that they have realistic expectations. Management of delayed healing may require revision of the amputation, aggressive wound care, and possibly conversion to a more proximal amputation level.

Postoperative infection

Controlling infection during the preoperative and postoperative periods is vital. In grossly infected cases, the amputation should be left open and be allowed to heal by secondary intention or delayed primary closure at a later date. An infectious disease consultation should be considered in infected cases. In the author's experience, most patients require a course of intravenous antibiotics during the perioperative period, then are converted to oral antibiotics until free of infection.

Summary

When distal amputations cannot be performed because of excessive soft tissue loss, one should consider a Lisfranc amputation. If combined with appropriate musculotendinous balancing procedures, this amputation level can provide a functional limb for ambulation and prevent a proximal amputation. Success with these amputations is reported to be 80% to 90% [4–9].

Chopart amputation

A more proximal midfoot amputation than Lisfranc amputation is one at Chopart's articulation. The disarticulation occurs through the talonavicular and calcaneocuboid joints. Only the talus and calcaneus are left of the foot. As with all amputations, a thorough workup has to be performed, especially when deciding if the proposed level of amputation will heal. A Chopart amputation also requires a viable heel pad.

The skin incision begins just proximal to the navicular tuberosity and extends dorsally between the fifth metatarsal base and lateral malleolus. Medial and lateral incisions extend distally along the first and fifth metatarsals. The midshafts of each incision are carried plantarly [10]. It is far easier to create too much of a plantar flap, which can be trimmed, than a flap that is too short. The flap is handled in an atraumatic fashion.

Usually the anterior process of the calcaneus and dorsal talar head are resected to eliminate bony prominences. Complete cartilage removal from the talus and calcaneus can lead to better flap adherence [11].

With the Chopart amputation, there is a great propensity for an equinovarus deformity to develop postoperatively [7,12]. This deformity can be avoided with an Achilles tendon tenotomy or lengthening combined with a transfer of the tibialis anterior into the lateral aspect of the talor neck fixated with the surgeon's preference. These ancillary procedures should be performed in every patient.

At University Hospital–UMDNJ, whenever an Achilles tendon needs to be lengthened because of a proximal amputation, a complete Achilles tenotomy is

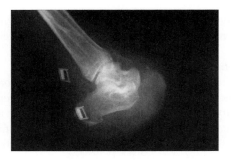

Fig. 5. Radiograph after Chopart amputation.

performed. A stab incision is made on either the medial or the lateral side of the Achilles tendon. The medial side is preferred because of the placement of the foot on the operating room table. It is easier to turn the foot so that the medial side is pointing toward the ceiling. The stab incision is at the Achilles tendon well away from the neurovascular bundle. Soft tissue is dissected from the anterior and posterior aspects of the Achilles using a blunt technique. A no. 15 blade is used to sever the tendon from anterior to posterior, with care being taken not to puncture the skin. As the incision is being made through the Achilles, the ankle is maximally dorsiflexed. One should hear the knife cutting the Achilles as if celery is being snapped, and once finished, the ankle should "give way" in a dorsiflexing direction. One or two skin sutures are all that is necessary to close this incision.

A drain is inserted at the surgeon's discretion. A posterior splint is applied with the foot in dorsiflexion. Under no circumstances should any tendon work be done in the presence of an infection. During the delayed closure, usually 3 to 7 days after the amputation, the tendon work is performed.

The residual stump after a Chopart amputation is short (Fig. 5). Minimally a custom-molded prosthesis is fabricated along with a rigid rubber-soled shoe [13]. A Chopart amputation, in contrast to the Symes, does leave enough of a stump that a minimal number of steps (ie, to the bathroom) can be taken without the prosthesis.

References

[1] Lis Franc J. Nouvelle methode operatoire pour l'amputation partielle dans so articulation tarsos-metatarsienne. Paris: Sabon; 1815.

[2] McDermott JE. The diabetic foot. American Academy of Orthopedic Surgeons Monograph series. Rosemont (IL): American Academy of Orthopedic Surgeons; 1995.

[3] Brodshy J. Transmetatarsal amputation. In: Master techniques in orthopedic surgery: the foot and ankle. New York: Raven Press; 1994. p. 213–27.

[4] Dickhaut SC, SeLee JC, Page CP. Nutritional status: importance in predicting wound healing after amputation. J Bone Joint Surg 1984;66A:71–5.

[5] Hobson MI, Stonebridge PA, Clason AE. Place of transmetatarsal amputations: a 5 year experience and review of the literature. J R Coll Surg Edinb 1990;35:113–5.

[6] Letts M, Pyper A. The modified Chopart's amputation. Clin Orthop 1990;256:44–9.

[7] Lieberman JR, Jacobs RI, Goldstock L, et al. Chopart amputation with percutaneous heel cord lengthening. Clin Orthop 1993;296:86–91.

[8] Patel KR, Chan FA, Clauss RH. Functional foot salvage after extensive plantar excision and amputations proximal to the standard metatarsal level. J Vasc Surg 1993;18:1030–6.

[9] Roach JJ, Deutsch A, McFarlane DS. Resections of the amputations of Lis franc and Chopart for diabetic gangrene. Arch Surg 1987;122:931–3.

[10] Sanders LJ. Transmetatarsal and midfoot amputations. Clin Podiatr Med Surg 1997;14:741–61.

[11] Chang BB, Bock DEM, Jacobs RL, et al. Increased limb salvage by the use of unconventional foot amputations. J Vasc Surg 1994;19:341–8.

[12] Early JS. Transmetatarsal and mid-foot amputations. Clin Orthop 1999;361:85–90.

[13] Bowker JH, San Giovanni TP. Amputations and disarticulations. In: Myerson MS, editor. Foot and ankle disorders. Philadelphia: WB Saunders; 2000. p. 466–503.

ELSEVIER
SAUNDERS

Clin Podiatr Med Surg
22 (2005) 395–427

CLINICS IN
PODIATRIC
MEDICINE AND
SURGERY

Syme's Amputation: A Retrospective Review of 10 Cases

Gerard V. Yu, DPM, FACFAS[a,b,]*, Theresa L. Schinke, DPM[a],
Amanda Meszaros, DPM[a]

[a]Section of Podiatry, Department of Surgery, St. Vincent Charity Hospital, Cleveland, OH, USA
[b]The Podiatry Institute, Tucker, GA, USA

Combined structural and functional preservation of the lower extremities is the goal of health care professionals dedicated to limb salvage in high-risk patients, especially the diabetic patient population, which continues to grow at an alarming rate. These goals are often unrealistic or unattainable because of a variety of pathologic conditions, most notably severe deformity and infectious processes in the soft tissue and bone recalcitrant to conservative treatment modalities. Critical limb ischemia further complicates some cases. When limb salvage is unrealistic, amputation may become the only realistic solution. Often a below-knee amputation or, more recently, a distal transtibial amputation is the outcome. This article discusses the value of the Syme's ankle disarticulation procedure as a potentially highly functional amputation with clear advantages and benefits over more proximal amputations.

In his original paper describing amputation at the level of the ankle joint in 1843, Syme expressed regret at the number of limbs that he previously had cut off that might have been saved with an alternative procedure [1]. This is a feeling shared by many foot and ankle surgeons whose patients have progressed to either a below-knee amputation or an above-knee amputation for conditions that were not amenable to either forefoot or midfoot amputations. At the time of its introduction, Syme's procedure was viewed as a major technical advance. The procedure was developed in the era before the advent of antiseptics and anesthesia, and one of Syme's major goals was to develop a safer and more reliable

---

* Corresponding author. 23823 Lorain Road, Suite 280, North Olmsted, OH 44070.
 E-mail address: gerardvyu@aol.com (G.V. Yu).

0891-8422/05/$ – see front matter © 2005 Elsevier Inc. All rights reserved.
doi:10.1016/j.cpm.2005.03.008 *podiatric.theclinics.com*

procedure than the traditional below-knee amputation, which at that time had a mortality rate of 25% to 50% [2].

Syme believed that compared with below-knee amputation, ankle amputation afforded a smaller risk of loss of life, a more comfortable stump, and a more useful limb for support and progressive motion [1]. Wagner popularized the procedure as a limb-salvage and function-sparing procedure [3]. He proposed a two-stage technique that he believed would decrease significantly the risk of infection and would ensure the preservation of the heel pad and distal tibia as entities for direct load transfer, more closely simulating normal weight bearing. He used Syme's procedure widely in patients with nonsalvageable infection or gangrene and, in an unpublished study, reported excellent results in more than 500 patients.

Today, more than 150 years after the introduction of Syme's amputation, the risk of death from sepsis or hemorrhage after a below-knee amputation is virtually zero, making Syme's amputation a safe procedure in the absence of comorbid conditions in a patient who is undergoing lower extremity amputation. Ankle amputation provides a more useful, durable stump that allows the amputee to function with little to no disability.

Periodic case reports in the literature have affirmed the long-term durability of this level of amputation with subjects enjoying more than 40 years of success with the stump [4,5]. More recent studies have shown a significant decrease in the energy and metabolic expenditures with ambulation experienced by patients who have undergone an ankle disarticulation procedure versus a higher transtibial amputation or even a more distal midfoot amputation, making Syme's procedure of even greater interest [4–8]. Current literature concerning morbidity and mortality shows that patients who have undergone a Syme's procedure experience less short-term morbidity and tend to survive longer overall compared with patients who have undergone a more proximal procedure [9]. Pinzur et al [10,20] observed that approximately 33% of patients who underwent a Syme's ankle disarticulation had died at 5 years postprocedure, whereas 33% of transtibial amputees died at 2 years postprocedure. The main advantages of Syme's procedure are a potentially fully weight-bearing stump of near-normal length, a swift and positive return to functional activity, and decreased mortality compared with transtibial amputation.

Despite these well-recognized advantages of the Syme's amputation, there has been a tendency toward its underuse; the procedure enjoys widespread popularity only in Canada and Scotland [2,6]. The reasons for underuse of Syme's amputation are multifactorial. Perhaps it is the perception that wound healing is routinely difficult and prolonged or that the residual stump is prone to ulceration or difficult to fit with a prosthesis. Perhaps it is the result of "tradition" that is passed on year in and year out with the established mindset being that a below-knee amputation is next in line after a failed midfoot amputation. The truth is that this procedure often is avoided simply because many foot and ankle surgeons have been indoctrinated with the notion that the procedure simply "does not work." As a consequence, more recently trained foot and ankle surgeons, whether orthopedic or podiatric, receive little, if any, training in the Syme's amputation procedure. The authors believe that many of the concerns regarding this procedure are ill-conceived misperceptions. The authors previously published a comprehensive review of the procedure, including a detailed description of the surgical technique. The senior author has continued to employ this procedure for a variety of foot and ankle conditions that traditionally would have required a higher level amputation; a retrospective review of cases is presented.

Surgical considerations

Syme's ankle disarticulation is indicated primarily in diabetic patients with gangrene, severe Charcot process, nonhealing dysvascular ulcers, and severe nonsalvageable diabetic foot infections; compromised arterial circulation is common. Syme's amputation may be used in any patient with a wide range of foot and ankle conditions, including congenital deformities, trauma/crush injury, soft tissue and osseous sarcomas of the foot, ischemia, frostbite, and osteomyelitis (Figs. 1–5).

Contraindications to performing a Syme's procedure include inadequate blood flow to the ankle and hind foot, infection or large open lesions of the heel pad, ascending cellulitis or lymphangitis, severe immunocompromise, or malnutrition. A lack of potential for the amputee to become a community ambulator after the procedure also should be considered a contraindication (Figs. 6 and 7) [9–11].

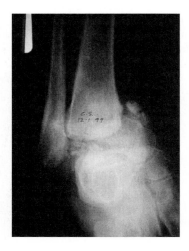

Fig. 1. Preoperative x-ray shows severe total collapse of the talus secondary to diabetic Charcot neuroarthropathy. The patient had been essentially wheelchair bound for approximately 1 year and developed ulceration over the fibular malleolus. Because of extensive comorbid conditions, including diabetes mellitus and blindness, amputation was recommended. The patient died several years after the amputation, but enjoyed improved quality of life during this time.

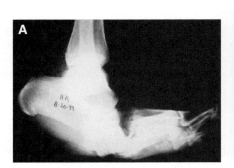

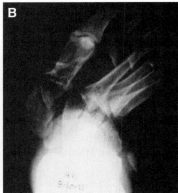

Fig. 2. (*A* and *B*) Preoperative radiographs reveal severe crush injury to the midfoot.

Healing of the amputation traditionally has not been problematic in patients undergoing the procedure for reasons other than severe peripheral vascular disease or diabetes-related manifestations. In cases in which the procedure is being performed for the latter entities, however, it is important to confirm the patient's healing capacity for this level of amputation; such requirements have been outlined by Wagner [3] and later modified by Dickhaut et al [12] and Pinzur et al [13,14].

Wound-healing parameters have been designed to predict whether the patient has the immunocompetence, nutritional status, and arterial inflow to heal the amputation (Table 1). Immunocompetence is predicted by an absolute lymphocyte count greater than $1500/mm^3$. The absolute lymphocyte count may be calculated by multiplying the total white blood cell count by the percentage of lymphocytes. A low total lymphocyte count may impair significantly a patient's

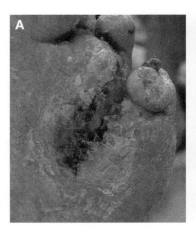

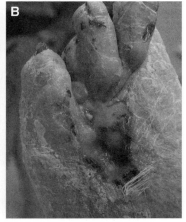

Fig. 3. (*A* and *B*) Clinical photographs reveal carcinoma localized to the forefoot.

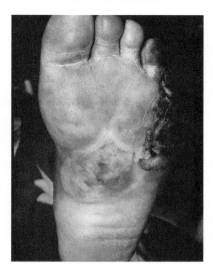

Fig. 4. Clinical appearance of a severe fetid foot with osteomyelitis. This patient underwent a two-stage procedure consisting of an incision and drainage with débridement followed by subsequent revision to a Syme's procedure. The postoperative recovery was unremarkable, and full ambulatory status was achieved.

risk to combat infection. A serum albumin level of greater than 3 g/dL (range 3.5–5 g/dL) and a total protein level of 6 g/dL or greater (range 6.4–8.3 g/dL) are required to ensure a minimal level of tissue nutrition. Neither serum albumin nor total protein levels should be used singly as indicators of nutritional competence. It has been shown that albumin and total protein levels are affected by hepatic and renal disease, overhydration, and underhydration and should be used as nutritional indicators only if used in conjunction with other markers [10,15,16]. Measuring the prealbumin level should be considered in all patients with a

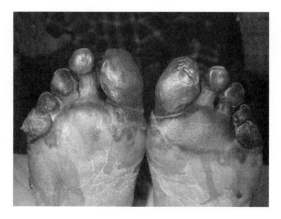

Fig. 5. Clinical photograph of severe frostbite to bilateral feet.

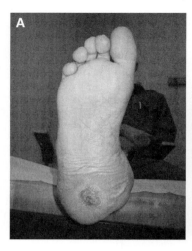

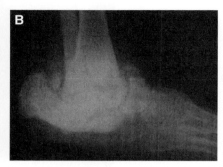

Fig. 6. Clinical (*A*) and radiographic (*B*) appearance of a patient with severe diabetes with multiple medical complications. The patient had sustained a severe diabetic plantar ulcer with chronic underlying osteomyelitis and underwent multiple surgeries. Complete atrophy of the plantar fat pad with adherence of the skin to the underlying bone was present, precluding the use of the plantar fat pad as the distal weight-bearing stump in the Syme's amputation.

borderline or questionable nutritional competence. Normal serum prealbumin level should be between 16 mg/dL and 35 mg/dL, and generally a level less than 10 mg/dL indicates moderate-to-severe nutritional deficiency. The prealbumin level generally is not influenced by external factors, and it provides an accurate representation of nutritional deficiency; it also can be used to monitor the effect

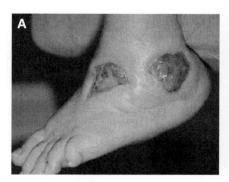

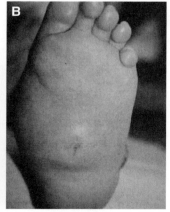

Fig. 7. (*A* and *B*) Clinical appearance of a patient with diabetic Charcot neuroarthropathy and chronic osteomyelitis. From the plantar perspective, it appears as if this patient may be a good candidate for a Syme's procedure. The presence of chronic ulcerations anteriorly and laterally secondary to peripheral vascular disease indicates, however, that the patient may be better served with a different procedure, such as a below-knee amputation.

Table 1
Preoperative requirements and predictors of success

Ankle-brachial index	> 0.5
Transcutaneous oxygen pressure	>30 mm Hg*
Total lymphocyte count	>1500/mm^3
Serum albumin level	>3 g/dL
Prealbumin level	>16–35 mg/dL
Serum glucose level	< 250 mg/dL
Highly motivated patient	
Access to a highly skilled prosthetist	

* Wound healing parameters for lower extremity amputations.

of dietary supplementation [10]. The authors recommend that all patients not meeting these minimal guidelines should undergo nutritional supplementation in the form of multivitamins, hyperalimentation of protein-rich foods, and arginine supplementation. Arginine has been shown to promote wound healing and increase the immune response by creating a positive nitrogen balance and enhancing T-lymphocyte function [17,18].

Optimal blood glucose levels should be maintained throughout the perioperative period to augment healing of the surgical wound further. After proper wound preparation, if antibiotic management of acute infectious processes and adjunctive nutritional measures have been implemented, and the patient fails to achieve the minimal recommended guidelines, a more proximal amputation might be warranted.

Adequate blood flow for healing is indicated by a palpable posterior tibial or dorsalis pedis pulse, an ankle-brachial index greater than 0.5, or a transcutaneous oxygen concentration of at least 30 mm Hg. The ankle-brachial index traditionally has been most useful in identifying patients who have disease of the macrocirculatory system and would benefit from some type of revascularization procedure before any planned amputation. The ankle-brachial index is not a direct reflection of tissue perfusion, however [19,20]. Ankle-brachial indices can be inadvertently elevated in the face of calcified vessels, making them difficult to occlude [13,14]. Measuring the transcutaneous oxygen tension may eliminate the concern of this variable.

Transcutaneous oxygen tension is measured through the application of superficially applied sensors on room air at multiple sites on the operative limb representing the various options for level of amputation (eg, the tibial crest, the anterior ankle, and the dorsal midfoot). The sensors directly measure the oxygen-delivering capacity or perfusion to the skin [13]. The general accepted value for healing an amputation site is greater than 30 mm Hg on room air [9,12,13,20]. Infected wounds pose an additional challenge, however, in that the increased bacterial load may suppress the transcutaneous oxygen tension value falsely secondary to increased oxygen consumption by macrophages and invading organisms [12,14,20]. Other considerations include operator error, proper device calibration, position of the limb, and room temperature. All of the aforementioned factors may compromise the validity of the measured transcutaneous oxygen tension values [14]. Some authors believe that careful control of such variables would improve diagnostic accuracy significantly, making the transcutaneous oxygen measurement the most valuable tool in preoperative screening [12,14,20].

Syme's amputation can be performed as either a one-stage or a two-stage procedure. In 1954, Spittler et al [21] described a two-stage approach to Syme's amputation that was performed for infected war wounds. In the first stage, the ankle joint was disarticulated, and "closure without tension" was performed. The second stage was performed 6 to 8 weeks later, at which time the malleoli were removed through medial and lateral elliptical incisions, and the wounds were closed. The rationale behind the two-stage procedure was to decrease the chance for infection after the procedure.

Wagner [3,33,34] was a proponent of the two-stage procedure in cases of severe diabetic foot infection. He reported close to a 95% success rate with the two-stage procedure when it was performed in patients who met the following clinical indications: positive potential for prosthetic use, heel pad free of open lesions, absence of pus at the amputation site, no ascending lymphangitis, and an ankle-brachial index greater than 0.45. Pinzur et al [22] evaluated the success of the two-stage procedure performed in diabetics with forefoot gangrene and nonreconstructible peripheral vascular disease. The results of the study revealed that 31 of 38 amputations eventually healed and were fitted with a prosthesis. Of the subjects, 27 (71%) eventually returned to their preamputation level of ambulatory function, providing significant testimony to the efficacy of this amputation.

In a later study, Pinzur et al [20,22,23] compared the results of the one-stage versus the two-stage Syme's procedure in patients undergoing amputation surgery for gangrene or nonsalvageable diabetic foot infections. The study was terminated early when the results from both procedures seemed to be similar. The authors concluded that the two-stage procedure subjected patients with high cardiac risk to a second hospitalization, anesthesia, and surgery, which resulted in higher overall health care costs. In that study, 44 one-stage and two-stage procedures were performed with 31 (70%) of the amputations progressing to wound healing and prosthesis fitting. In 2003, Pinzur et al [38] presented a study that illustrated an 88% overall success rate when all parameters for adequate vascular inflow and tissue nutrition were met. In the same study, they further explored the role of the total lymphocyte count in wound healing and found that neither a low lymphocyte count nor smoking significantly impaired the rate of wound healing, yet smoking did contribute significantly to an infection rate three times that of nonsmokers [38].

Although the two-stage procedure is useful in cases with aggressive soft tissue infection, the one-stage procedure is more commonly employed. Typically the one-stage procedure employs a fish-mouth incision about the ankle joint that preserves the plantar heel pad and allows for the disarticulation of the ankle joint and resection of the malleoli. One of the most important criteria for performing this procedure is the presence of a viable plantar heel pad because this is the ultimate weight-bearing interface between the tibia/fibula and prosthetic device.

The plantar fat pad is composed of a meshwork of fat that is enclosed within fibroelastic septa arranged in a closed-cell configuration [24]. This unique anatomic configuration allows the plantar fat pad to function as a shock-absorbing structure during ambulation. Given its importance in pain-free weight bearing, every effort must be made to maintain the structural integrity of the plantar fat pad during a Syme's procedure; this is best accomplished by employing subperiosteal dissection whenever possible when removing the calcaneus.

Various modifications to the standard incisional approach, including an anterior ankle flap for use in patients in whom it is not possible to use the heel as a flap, have been described [25]. Although the anterior flap may provide adequate soft tissue coverage for an ankle amputation in which the heel pad is nonviable, the anterior flap does not contain the same shock-absorbing qualities as the plantar fat pad and may result in an uncomfortable stump, eliminating a favorable aspect of the Syme's amputation (Fig. 8).

Postoperatively the first several weeks are crucial for Syme's amputation. During this time, the wound is most at risk for dehiscence, slough, or other related complications. Hematoma and seroma formation are common occurrences and must be managed appropriately. Meticulous hemostasis and the use of a surgical drain are important considerations. In addition, wound healing complications can be lessened by employing an atraumatic surgical technique; gentle tissue handling is essential for success. Inadvertent transection of the posterior tibial artery proximal to the distal aspect of the plantar flap also may compromise healing in the early days after the procedure. Provided that vascularity is maintained in the flap, predictable stability of the wound is typical after healing of the

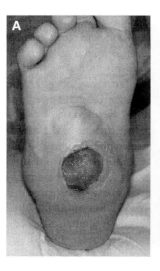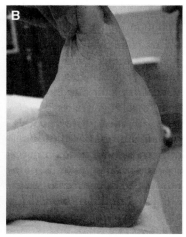

Fig. 8. (*A* and *B*) Preoperative clinical photographs of a chronic ulceration with underlying severe osteomyelitis of 2 years' duration. In planning for consideration of a Syme's amputation, an adequate heel pad must be present, providing coverage and support. A more proximal ulcer would be considered a relative contraindication to the Syme's procedure.

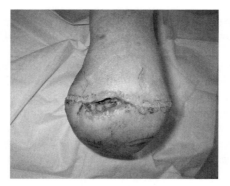

Fig. 9. Postoperative wound complication after Syme's amputation in a patient with chronic underlying osteomyelitis. The patient was returned to the operating room for débridement and drainage with subsequent closure. The patient went on to heal the wound successfully.

initial incision (Figs. 9 and 10). Late complications also may occur, including hypermobility and improper location of the plantar fat pad, stump sensitivity, neuroma formation, and phantom pain. These complications are not unique to this type of amputation and are associated with amputations in general (Figs. 11 and 12).

Surgical technique

The surgical procedure is performed with the patient in a supine position. A calf or thigh pneumatic tourniquet is used if no contraindications are present. A modified fish-mouth incision that preserves the plantar fat pad is outlined about the ankle joint. The key landmarks for creating this flap are the inferior aspects of the malleoli. A point 1 cm inferior and 1 cm anterior to the tip of the lateral malleolus is marked. Next, a point 1.5 cm inferior and 1 cm anterior to the tip of

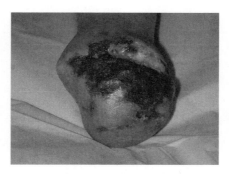

Fig. 10. Failed clinical appearance of a wound after Syme's amputation performed elsewhere in a patient with inadequate arterial perfusion. Appropriate preoperative screening and vascular assessment could have precluded this unfortunate outcome. A below-knee amputation was the final outcome.

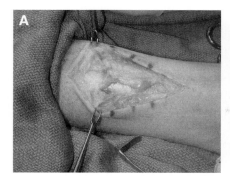
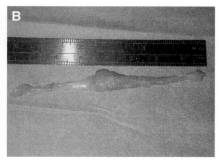

Fig. 11. (*A* and *B*) Intraoperative photograph shows recurrent stump neuroma after Syme's amputation in a non-neuropathic patient. The patient underwent a Syme's amputation after a severe crush injury to the foot.

the medial malleolus is marked. These points are connected with a line drawn crossing the anterior aspect of the ankle; it is important that the incision is not proximal to the distal aspect of the tibia. The plantar incision is oriented approximately 90° from the dorsal incision and drawn out across the plantar surface of the foot extending from the two points below the malleoli. The plantar incision should be performed to the level of the calcaneocuboid joint to ensure adequate length of the plantar flap. When designing this flap, it is better to err on the side of too long a flap, which always can be modified before skin closure. Proper planning of the skin incision cannot be overemphasized. Visualization of the final desired product is a necessary prerequisite for success (Fig. 13).

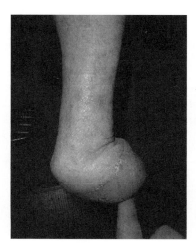

Fig. 12. Postoperative appearance of an excessively mobile stump. A revisional procedure was performed to anchor the stump adequately.

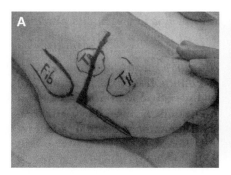
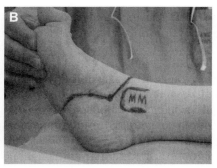

Fig. 13. (*A* and *B*) Preoperative incision planning for Syme's amputation. Note the relationship of the incisions to the malleoli and preservation of the plantar heel pad. The anterior incision is distal to the tibial plafond.

Although the skin incisions may be made directly to bone, the authors prefer making a controlled-depth incision. With this approach, improved hemostasis and anatomic dissection are achieved. The anterior incision is performed first. No undermining of the incision is performed. Dissection is carried down through the subcutaneous tissue to the level of the deep fascia. Superficial nerves crossing the anterior ankle joint (saphenous, medial, and intermediate dorsal cutaneous nerves) are identified, pulled distally, sharply transected, and allowed to migrate proximally. All superficial veins are ligated or cauterized as necessary. The deep fascia is incised, and the anterior tendons crossing the ankle joint are identified, clamped, pulled distally, sharply transected, and allowed to migrate proximally; these include the tibialis anterior, the extensor hallucis longus, the extensor digitorum longus, and, if present, the peroneus tertius. The anterior tibial artery is identified and ligated. The deep peroneal nerve is cut under traction and allowed to migrate proximally as well. The anterior ankle joint capsule is now exposed (Fig. 14).

The plantar incision is developed next. The use of a controlled-depth incision without undermining is recommended. The incision is deepened through the

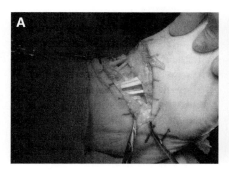
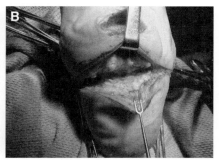

Fig. 14. Intraoperative appearance of the anterior incision (*A*) with the anterior tendons exposed and the plantar incision (*B*).

subcutaneous tissues of the plantar foot. The lateral dorsal cutaneous nerve is cut under traction and allowed to retract proximally, as is the lesser saphenous vein after ligation. The peroneal tendons are identified, placed under traction, severed, and allowed to retract proximally. Dissection of the plantar flap is complete at this point when the plantar fascia is visualized. There should be no dissection along the plane of the plantar fascia.

Attention is redirected to the anterior aspect of the ankle joint, and the capsule is incised. The dome of the talus is now visualized. Transecting the medial and lateral ankle ligaments from the talus allows disarticulation of the ankle joint. Great care must be taken when transecting the medial collateral ligaments to avoid inadvertent transection of the posterior tibial artery, veins, and nerve that lie in close proximity. Preservation of the artery at its maximal length is imperative because it is the primary blood supply to the plantar flap. The long flexor tendons and the posterior tibial tendon are isolated, placed under distal traction, transected, and allowed to migrate proximally. At this point, blunt dissection of the posterior tibial neurovascular bundle should be performed to isolate this structure in the posterior flap. The posterior tibial artery should be traced as far distally as possible and ligated. Next, the posterior tibial nerve is cut under tension and allowed to migrate proximally.

The foot is plantar flexed, and the posterior ankle joint capsule and periarticular structures are transected. Placing a bone hook into the posterior aspect of the talus and applying distal traction allows increased exposure to the posterior aspect of the ankle joint. The insertion of the Achilles tendon is identified and released from the calcaneus. There is little subcutaneous tissue between the Achilles tendon and posterior skin. The authors encourage meticulous sharp dissection technique in this area to prevent buttonholing. A Crego elevator may be a safer and more useful instrument for freeing the insertion of the Achilles tendon. After transection of the tendon, further plantar flexion of the foot allows subperiosteal dissection of the posterior, medial, lateral, and plantar surfaces of the calcaneus from its underlying soft tissue attachments. At this point, the remaining insertions of the plantar fascia and intrinsic musculature to the calcaneus are transected, and the foot is delivered from the operative field.

Occasionally the authors have found it advantageous to disarticulate the foot at Chopart's joint before removing the talus and calcaneus from the ankle joint. After removal of the distal foot, large threaded Steinmann pins are driven into the head of the talus and the distal articular surface of the calcaneus. These pins are used as "joysticks" to facilitate subperiosteal dissection of the calcaneus or talus.

When the entire foot has been removed, attention is directed toward the resection of the tibia and fibula. The articular cartilage of the distal tibia may be retained or resected. Removal of the articular cartilage from the distal tibia may allow for better adherence of the plantar fat pad postoperatively, but contributes to increased limb shortening. In cases of severe infection in which spread to the tibia is of concern, the cartilage at the distal end of the tibia may be left intact to serve as a physical barrier to the spread of bacteria. Resection is accomplished with a large power saw placed perpendicular to the long axis of the tibia and

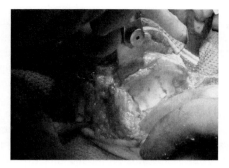

Fig. 15. Intraoperative photograph of resection of the articular cartilage at the distal tibia. Resection can be accomplished using a large power saw. The bone cuts should be made parallel to the ground supporting surface, taking care to preserve as much of the distal tibia as possible.

fibula. The bone cuts are made parallel to the ground-supporting surface of the distal tibia. Care is taken to preserve as much of the distal tibia as possible to maintain a large weight-bearing surface area. Further remodeling of the distal end of the tibia and fibula is required to square off the osseous component of the stump. The medial and lateral malleoli are resected at a 45° to 60° angle from the long axis from their respective bones, creating a narrow distal stump, which facilitates an optimal fit of the prosthesis (Fig. 15).

Before closure, drill holes can be made along the distal anterior and distal posterior aspect of the tibia, and the Achilles tendon and other remaining deep soft tissues can be secured with nonabsorbable suture. Tenodesis of the Achilles tendon to the tibia has been shown to an effective method for decreasing mobility and maintaining the position of the fat pad at the end of the osseous stump (Fig. 16) [26].

If a tourniquet is used, it is deflated at this time, and additional hemostasis is achieved as necessary; although smaller vessels respond well to electrocoagulation, larger lumen vessels should be ligated. A large-lumen, closed-suction

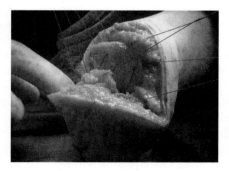

Fig. 16. Intraoperative photograph shows several drill holes in the distal tibia after resection of the articular surface and malleoli. Nonabsorbable suture is used to secure the distal aspect of the plantar fascia to the tibia to decrease mobility of the stump.

drain is introduced through a separate stab incision and placed within the surgical site. The deep fascia and residual collateral ligamentous tissues are reapproximated over the remaining bone with absorbable synthetic suture of choice.

At this time, the plantar flap is advanced, and debulking of the residual intrinsic musculature is performed as necessary. The subcutaneous tissues are reapproximated, and the skin is closed with either simple interrupted sutures of 3-0 synthetic monofilament nonabsorbable suture of choice or, if preferred, skin staples. Subcuticular closure of the skin is not recommended. It is common for "dog ears" to be present on the medial and lateral aspects of the incision. These can be remodeled, but must be done cautiously. It is common to allow these dog ears simply to remodel with time on their own accord or to return to the operating room for scar revision if needed. Pinzur [27] suggested that the creation of dog ears may be avoided by placing the apex of the incision just anterior and inferior to the midpoint of the medial and lateral malleoli. The authors have not found dog ears to be a significant problem (Fig. 17).

Initially the wound is dressed in a well-molded modified Jones compression bandage to minimize edema and hematoma or seroma formation; this dressing also helps to "contour" the stump as the tissues shrink and adapt. The patient is maintained non–weight bearing for 3 to 6 weeks until the wound has completely healed; sutures generally are removed around 2 to 4 weeks postoperatively. At that time, the patient can be placed in a short leg cast, and weight bearing as tolerated is permitted. The cast is changed at 2- to 3-week intervals until resolution of all soft tissue edema and stump shrinkage has occurred (Fig. 18). By approximately 5 to 9 weeks, the stump has stabilized, and the patient is referred to a prosthetist for the fabrication of a preparatory prosthetic device. The preparatory device is used for 3 to 9 months or until shaping and volumetric stabilization of the stump has occurred [38]. At that time, the patient is ready for the fabrication of a permanent prosthetic device (Fig. 19).

Physical therapy with the prosthesis in place is employed as necessary. In general, it has been the authors' experience that only minimal gait training is required. This need for only minimal training is mainly due to the length of the limb that is maintained. It also is partly due to the fact that the heel pad has been

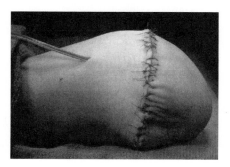

Fig. 17. Final appearance of the amputation site with drain in place.

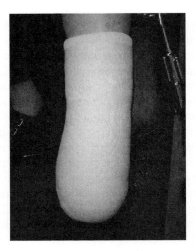

Fig. 18. Temporary fiberglass case used before obtaining a temporary prosthesis. This cast is applied at approximately 2 to 4 weeks postoperatively after removal of the sutures. Weight bearing is allowed as tolerated.

preserved, however, with some maintenance of normal proprioceptive pathways. Short periods of ambulation without the prosthesis, such as getting up to go to the bathroom in the middle of the night, are possible, although the limb-length discrepancy may hinder ambulation.

Prosthetic considerations

The prosthetic management of the Syme's level amputee must encompass several objectives. The prosthesis should compensate for the loss of foot and ankle motion, while providing the propulsive energy required for ambulation. It also is necessary to compensate for the limb-length discrepancy created by this

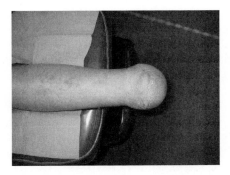

Fig. 19. Clinical presentation of a well-healed stump after Syme's amputation. Note the presence of the plantar heel pad for shock absorption. The distal stump is extremely durable.

level of amputation and to suspend the prosthesis adequately during swing phase of gait. This level of amputation has many functional advantages, but also has some prosthetic component limitations and cosmetic limitations resulting from the nature and shape of the residual limb being managed.

Biomechanically the prosthesis must be aligned to enhance gait while minimizing shear and providing a comfortable transition of forces to the residual limb. The prosthetist works to align the prosthetic foot as far posterior as cosmetically acceptable, with slight dorsiflexion, to minimize knee extension forces from midstance to toe-off phases of gait. In the coronal plane, the foot is placed lateral to the midline of the limb to provide medial-to-lateral stability. Slight eversion allows the foot to be flat on the ground at midstance. In the transverse plane, the foot is generally externally rotated as much as cosmetically acceptable to minimize knee extension forces at toe-off and provide medial-to-lateral stability by widening the base of support [28,32].

There are four basic designs of prostheses that currently are used in managing the Syme's level amputee. The posterior door design, also known as the Canadian design, is more commonly used on patients with large or bulbous residual limbs and is used frequently with Chopart's amputations. This design is ordered least often because it is the least cosmetic and has a heavier weight as a result of its construction parameters [29].

The most frequently used design is the medial opening or medial door design (Fig. 20). This design has great suspension characteristics as a result of the intimate nature of the socket construction. An elastic sleeve placed over the door improves cosmesis and facilitates the donning and doffing process by allowing the door to expand [30].

Another design employs the use of an expandable inner liner enclosed within the rigid outer shell. This design allows for the distal end of the stump to pass through expandable bladder portion. This hidden panel expandable wall design is indicated for patients with small distal ends and is considered the most cosmetic of all designs [31].

The fourth and final design often used for the preparatory prosthesis is one that uses a removable foam liner that interfaces with the external socket. This removable liner offers the prosthetist the ability to modify the insert to allow for the atrophy that occurs in the limb during the maturation process. This design offers great cosmesis, is lightweight in construction, and is highly adjustable. The medial door, hidden panel, and removable foam liner designs are best used on residual limbs that have had the malleoli removed for optimal reduction of distal end size.

Because of the length of the residual limb, prosthetic management has limitations in the number of prosthetic feet available (see Fig. 20). Traditionally, standard solid ankle cushion heel feet were employed in preparatory Syme's prosthesis because weight and biomechanical objectives were well served with this foot. Geriatric and low-level ambulators are still well served with this foot construction. There has been a resurgence in the development of energy-storing or dynamic feet for the Syme's prosthesis, which offer decreased weight and

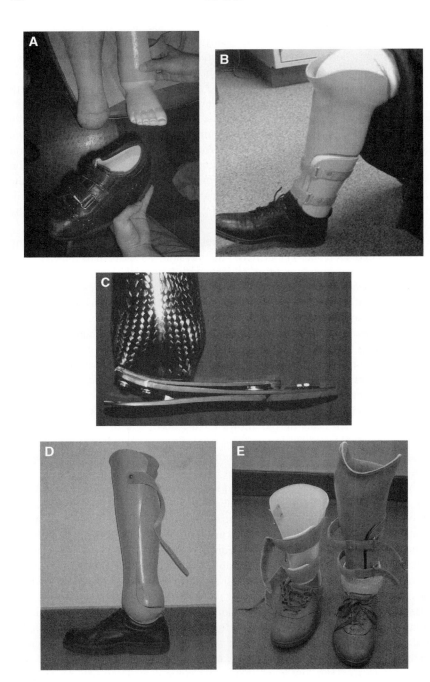

Fig. 20. (*A–F*) Prosthetic designs. The prosthesis must compensate for loss of foot and ankle motion and provide the propulsion energy necessary for ambulation.

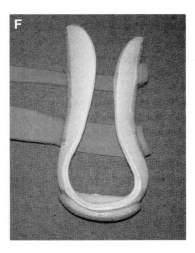

Fig. 20 (*continued*).

enhanced performance for the amputee. These prosthetic feet best serve amputees who will challenge the limits of prosthetic use.

The investigation into the success of Syme's amputation has led several authors to explore whether an ankle disarticulation truly leaves the patient with a more functional and efficient limb compared with more proximal levels of amputation. Pinzur et al [35] discovered that cadence and normal walking speed were impaired as the level of amputation extended more proximally. In addition, the rate of oxygen consumption and cardiac stress also increased with more proximal amputations. This is an important consideration given that much of the involved patient population has preexisting cardiovascular disease, and that an amputation at any level creates new demands on the system as a whole, most notably the cardiac and respiratory systems [7,8,32,33,36,37]. Devices such as canes, walkers, and crutches may offer the patient assistance and stability during ambulation; however, they negatively affect oxygen consumption, heart rate, and energy expenditure because of the arm movements and strength required to use such devices [7,8,32,33,36,37]. Careful consideration is necessary when planning the postoperative course of weight bearing and prosthetic management in high-risk individuals.

From a prosthetic management prospective, it is the authors' opinion that the advantages of the Syme's amputation far outweigh most, if not all, of its disadvantages. Advantages include decreased energy expenditure, more normal gait, and increased residual limb surface area to transfer and absorb socket pressures [28,32]. The disadvantages of the cosmetic appearance of the prosthesis and migration of the heel pad in some are minor in comparison [30].

Syme's amputations are a viable, highly successful level of amputation to consider for patients who meet the preoperative indications. Surgeons would be well advised to seek out the opinion of a prosthetist, preferably preoperatively whenever possible, to establish a prosthetic opinion and to help the future amputee feel more comfortable with the procedure and process. It is advisable to have the potential amputee see and feel a prosthesis, meet the bracemaker, and talk to an experienced Syme's amputee before moving forward with the amputation. The surgeon-prosthetist relationship can enhance outcomes by combining the talents of both and increasing the confidence and comfort level of the patient. Amputee support groups can be a valuable adjunct in the management of these patients.

Case Studies

Case 1

This patient was a 51-year-old woman admitted to our institution with a 20-year history of type 1 diabetes with multiple diabetic complications, including neuropathy, retinopathy, nephropathy, and cardiopathy, and gastroesophageal reflux disorder and hypercholesterolemia. She had a complicated history of pedal problems, including multiple surgeries of both feet with multiple hallux and digital amputations and partial ray resections. Her current problem consisted of a large chronic, nonhealing ulcer with associated sinus tract and underlying chronic tarsal osteomyelitis caused primarily by methicillin-resistant *Staphylococcus aureus*. She had been treated unsuccessfully parenterally for 6 months with vancomycin, ticarcillin-clavulanate, and ciprofloxacin. Previous attempts at periodic débridement proved unsuccessful, and the patient had been essentially wheelchair bound for several months before referral to the authors' institution.

The patient was considered to be a poor candidate for post–below-knee amputation rehabilitation because of her prior history of myocardial infarction, ischemic heart disease, and multiple comorbid conditions. She was taking numerous medications for diabetes. Physical examination revealed morbid obesity with stable vital signs. A large 2.5-cm cone-shaped ulceration was present on the left foot with granulation tissue and a deep sinus tract. Exuberant serous drainage was present. Multiple digits were missing as a result of prior amputations. Post-surgical scars also were noted. There were no open wounds present on the right foot. Her white blood cell count was 11,000/mm^3 on admission. Remaining laboratory studies were normal. Noninvasive vascular studies revealed tibial vessel occlusive disease, although digital photoplethysmography suggested adequate perfusion for healing (Fig. 21).

Pedal radiographs correlated with clinical observations, showing multiple digital amputations and severe bony destruction. These findings were consistent with Charcot neuroarthropathy with a superimposed chronic osteomyelitis (Fig. 22).

Reconstructive surgery was not considered a realistic option. Previous recommendations were for below-knee amputation. Given her significant medical history, however, it was thought that a pedal amputation would be more appropriate

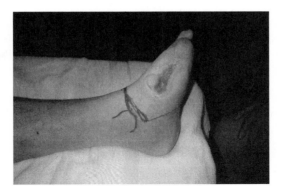

Fig. 21. Preoperative clinical photograph of a chronic wound of the left foot. The patient has undergone multiple previous surgeries for débridement and partial amputations unsuccessfully.

with less compromise to her cardiorespiratory function. The patient readily accepted an option of Syme's amputation in lieu of a below-knee amputation. Prophylactic bracing with a custom ankle-foot orthosis and extra-depth shoe was instituted for her contralateral extremity. In December 2002, she underwent a Syme's amputation under general anesthesia without immediate postoperative complications. Final pathology report was consistent with chronic ulceration, sinus tract formation, and extensive acute and chronic osteomyelitis. Atherosclerosis and calcification of the medium-sized arteries also were noted. She went on to successful uneventful healing of the surgical site without complication. The patient was fitted with a temporary prosthesis at approximately 6 weeks after surgery, but experienced several prosthetic complications, including ill fit and back pain secondary to a persistent limb-length discrepancy. After several ad-

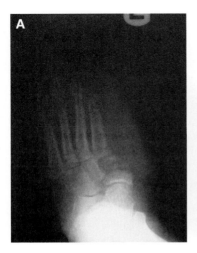

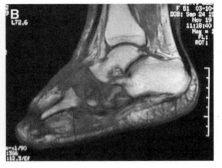

Fig. 22. (A) Preoperative x-ray shows prior surgical resection with extensive chronic osteomyelitis extending into the tarsus and metatarsal bases of the foot. (B) MRI confirmed osteomyelitis.

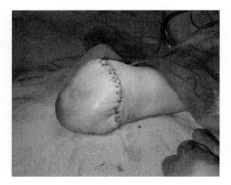

Fig. 23. Intraoperative appearance after completion of the Syme's procedure and closure of the wound. Uneventful healing occurred. No further extension of the osteomyelitis occurred.

justments, she became fully ambulatory without gait assistive devices at approximately 1 year postoperatively (Figs. 23 and 24).

Case 2

This patient was a 52-year-old man with past medical history of type 2 diabetes mellitus for 2 years, diabetic neuropathy, hypertension, and hypothyroidism. On initial presentation, the patient related a 1-year history of redness and swelling about the right foot and leg, but was not recognized as having an acute Charcot process until presentation to the authors' institution in mid-2003. The delay in proper treatment resulted in significant pedal collapse and loss of structural integrity. The patient had multiple pedal complications beginning with

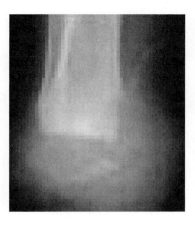

Fig. 24. After completion of Syme's amputation, note the tapering and configuration of the distal stump with resection of the malleoli.

a deep abscess, which resulted in an extensive incision and drainage of the plantar foot in early 2003. Postoperative wound cultures revealed methicillin-resistant *S. aureus*. The patient also underwent a third digit amputation of the same foot.

At the time of presentation, the patient was taking multiple medications for his several medical conditions. Physical examination revealed a morbidly obese man with stable vital signs. There was a hypergranular, full-thickness deep ulceration on the plantar aspect of the right foot measuring 5 × 6 cm in diameter with a large amount of serous drainage. The wound probed directly to bone. Conventional pedal radiographs, CT scans, indium scanning, and bone biopsy confirmed the presence of widespread osteomyelitis of the tarsal bones (Fig. 25).

Syme's amputation was recommended to provide the patient with the best functional outcome and to minimize strain on the cardiovascular and respiratory systems. He was fully amenable to amputation and underwent a Syme's amputation in September 2003. The patient had a minor postoperative infection and wound dehiscence. A second surgery consisting of wound débridement and scar revision was performed approximately 1 month later. The patient went on to heal completely and was fitted with a temporary prosthesis in November 2003. He has since been fitted with a permanent prosthesis and has no functional limitations to date. He is pleased with his prosthesis and his current level of function (Figs. 26 and 27).

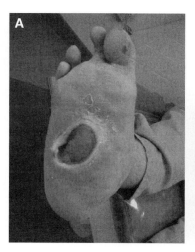
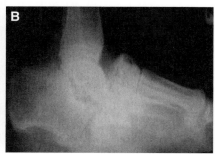

Fig. 25. Preoperative clinical appearance (*A*) and lateral radiograph (*B*) show severe plantar ulceration secondary to underlying diabetic Charcot neuroarthropathy with total collapse and fragmentation of the midtarsus and long-standing chronic osteomyelitis. The patient has had extensive long-term care without success and multiple bouts of oral and parenteral antibiotics.

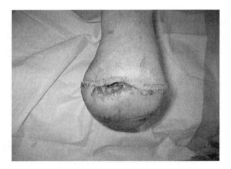

Fig. 26. Postoperative wound dehiscence necessitating revision, including excision of the lesion and primary closure. The patient subsequently healed with further local wound care.

Case 3

This patient was a 52-year-old man who presented to the office complaining of severe right clubfoot deformity since birth. Correction via posteromedial release had been attempted at age 15 but was unsuccessful, and the deformity had continued to progress. The patient had been treated with a Charcot Restraint Orthotic Walker device but had chronic irritation and pain despite multiple adjustments and alterations. His symptoms were aggravated with ambulation, and he complained specifically of instability and loss of balance while walking. He had a past medical history of spastic cerebral palsy, mitral regurgitation, obsessive-compulsive disorder, and hypertension. His current medications included citalopram (Celexa) and bupropion (Wellbutrin). The patient was unemployed and on disability; he had strong familial support at home.

Initial physical examination revealed that the right foot was in severe equinus, adduction, and varus malalignment. Overall the foot was found to be quite rigid with significant fixed contractures of the medial tendons and ligaments compounded by contracture of the overlying skin. Severe muscle and soft tissue atrophy and severe digital deformities with complete dislocations at all of the

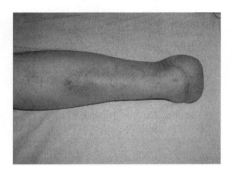

Fig. 27. The final appearance of the stump after compete healing. No further breakdown or wound complications were experienced. The patient resumed full activities of daily living.

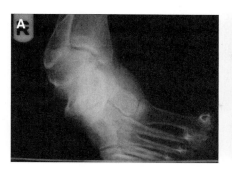
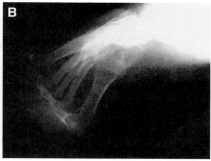

Fig. 28. Weight-bearing preoperative radiographs of the ankle (*A*) and foot (*B*) show severe fixed deformity with joint dislocation. Previous surgical intervention failed. The patient had poor skin integrity overlying the medial aspect of the foot and ankle.

metatarsophalangeal joints were found. Radiographs confirmed a complete medial subtalar and midtarsal joint dislocation and a ball-and-socket ankle joint with significant adaptive changes throughout (Fig. 28).

Several options for staged surgical treatment were offered, including pantalar arthrodesis with probable talectomy followed by relocation arthrodesis of the hallux and lesser toes with a probable first metatarsal osteotomy. After explaining the high likelihood of medial wound complications and the prolonged recovery and convalescence period after this multistage reconstructive surgery, the patient and family expressed a major concern over his physical, mental, and emotional limitations and his probable inability to remain non–weight bearing for any significant period because of mental impairment. Previous consultations with an orthopedic surgeon resulted in a strong recommendation for below-knee amputation. Multiple consultations with the patient and family occurred. The option

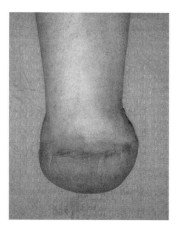

Fig. 29. Final clinical appearance of the stump after successful uncomplicated healing. The patient resumed full weight-bearing activities and was extremely pleased with the final outcome.

Table 2
Review of 10 cases

Sex	Age	Comorbid conditions	Additional considerations	Reason for amputation	DOS	Healing complications
M	52	IDDM, HTN, morbid obesity, hypothyroidism	Patient not desirous of keeping limb, desired a return to daily activity	Previously undiagnosed Charcot, chronic ulcer with widespread underlying osteomyelitis of the tarsal bones	9.29.2003	Minor postoperative infection and wound dehiscence, débridement 1 mo postoperative
F	51	IDDM, neuropathy, retinopathy, GERD, nephropathy, cardiopathy, hypercholesterolemia	Prior MI, ischemic heart disease	Severe Charcot arthropathy, chronic ulcer with underlying chronic osteomyelitis	12.02.2002	Minor wound dehiscence, knee irritation secondary to ill-fitting prosthesis
M	51	CP, HTN, mitral regurgitation	Slight mental deficit, patient not committed to long-term convalescence	Severe rigid nonreducible clubfoot deformity secondary to spastic CP with overlying compromised skin	1.28.2002	None
M	52	ESRD, IDDM, HTN, CAD, hypothyroidism	Difficulty with NWB, patient not committed to long-term convalescence required for reconstruction	Severe Charcot arthropathy with multiple joint involvement	10.30.2003	None
M	22	None	Patient is young, healthy, wishes to preserve as much of the limb as possible	Severe trauma, crush injury resulting in traumatic forefoot amputation	9.3.1999	Stump neuroma × 3
F	76	RA, HTN, hypothyroidism, AAA	Difficulty with NWB secondary to RA	Nonhealing wound with chronic underlying osteomyelitis, squamous cell carcinoma	8.20.2001	Wound dehiscence, small, stump revision 2 to hypermobility

Sex	Age					
M	47	IDDM × 19 y, hypercholesterolemia, sleep apnea, HTN, vestibular dysfunction	Obesity	Charcot arthropathy with widespread joint destruction, chronic osetomyelitis	1.27.2003	Small central wound dehiscence, small central wound secondary to ill-fitting temporary prosthesis
F	65	IDDM × 25 y, HTN, CVA	Noncompliant with NWB	Severe midfoot Charcot with diffuse osseous destruction	7.19.2001	None
F	36	IDDM, CRI, retinopathy	Long-term immunosuppressive therapy secondary to kidney-pancreas transplant 7 y earlier, patient had been wheelchair bound for 2 y, was not desirous of additional attempts at salvage	Severe Charcot with varus dislocation, unsuccessful bracing attempts left patient wheelchair bound	3.15.2000	Wound dehiscence at 7 wk, revisional surgery at 8 and 16 weeks
M	52	Uncontrolled NIDDM	Admits to noncompliance in the past	Extensive deep space infection with osteomyelitis of multiple metatarsals and extension into arch	7.12.2000	None

Abbreviations: AAA, abdominal aortic aneurysm; CAD, coronary artery disease; CP, cerebral palsy; CRI, chronic renal insufficiency; CVA, cerebrovascular accident; ESRD, end-stage renal disease; GERD, gastroesophageal reflux disease; HTN, hypertension; IDDM, insulin-dependent diabetes mellitus; NWB, non–weight bearing; RA, rheumatoid arthritis.

of a Syme's amputation was offered. The patient and family were amenable to amputation and decided to proceed with a Syme's disarticulation with the hope of attaining a quick return to full function without gait-assistive devices and to relieve pain (Fig. 29).

The patient underwent a Syme's ankle disarticulation procedure in January 2002. He had an uneventful postoperative course, and the surgical site healed successfully. He was fitted with a temporary prosthesis in April 2002 and progressed to full weight bearing without assistive devices and no functional limitations. He has been appreciative of his markedly improved quality of life and frequently refers to the prosthesis as his "new foot."

Results

A retrospective review of 10 cases performed at the authors' institution between 1999 and 2003 was conducted (Table 2). Of the 10 patients, 4 were women, and 6 were men, with an average age of 50.4 years (range 22–76 years). Comorbid conditions included diabetes mellitus ($n = 7$), hypertension ($n = 6$), end-stage renal disease ($n = 2$), rheumatoid arthritis ($n = 1$), morbid obesity ($n = 2$), coronary artery disease ($n = 2$), and hypercholesterolemia ($n = 3$). One patient had undergone a pancreas and kidney transplant 7 years earlier, and a second was status post cerebrovascular accident 8 years previously. Additional complicating factors included noncompliance with prior care and mental handicap secondary to cerebral palsy.

Of the 10 patients studied, 6 underwent a Syme's amputation secondary to severe Charcot neuroarthropathy with or without underlying osteomyelitis; 1 patient had a nonsalvageable foot secondary to deep space infection and osteomyelitis; 1 patient had osteomyelitis and squamous cell carcinoma underlying a chronic, nonhealing wound; 1 patient had a severe crush injury and traumatic amputation at the midfoot; and 1 patient had a painful rigid severe clubfoot deformity secondary to spastic cerebral palsy. All patients had successful healing of the surgical site, and none of the patients progressed to a higher level amputation.

The most common postoperative complication was wound dehiscence, which occurred in five patients. Two patients required wound débridement or stump revision. One patient required revisional surgery because of a hypermobile stump. Another common postoperative complication involved an ill-fitting prosthesis. Two patients developed minor wounds secondary to their ill-fitting prosthesis; three additional patients complained of a loose device, a heavy device, or unstable foot prostheses. The average length of time before each patient was fitted with a temporary prosthesis was 10 weeks. One patient did not become ambulatory for 1.5 years because of an active contralateral Charcot process. Each of the remaining patients became fully ambulatory in a permanent prosthesis without gait assistive devices 4 to 6 months postoperatively.

Table 3
Follow-up study

Sex	Age	Temporary prosthesis	Permanent prosthesis	Activity level
M	52	11.2003 (5 wk postop)	3.04 y	Full WB without limitation, increased activity compared with preoperatively
F	51	6 wk postop		Progressed to full WB, able to perform activities of daily living without assistance
M	51	3.2002 (6 wk postop)	8.02 y	Full WB, increased activity without pain, uses cane to assist over long distances
M	52			Full WB, minor difficulty walking uphill
M	22			Returned to work, full activity
F	76	10.4.01(6.5 wk postop)		Difficulty ambulating in prosthesis, heavy
M	47	3.12.03 (6 wk postop)		Full WB 8 wk postop, lost to follow-up
F	65	8.20.01 (4 wk postop)		No restrictions, cleared from PT on 9/20/01
F	36	1.5 y postop secondary to contralateral Charcot		Full activity without additional assistive devices, patient died 2 y postop due to diabetic complications
M	52	9.12.00 (8 wk postop)	6 mo	Full activity with minimal disability

Overall, long-term follow-up was encouraging, with seven patients relaying improved quality of life postoperatively and ability to perform activities of daily living without limitation or assistance (Table 3). Two patients were lost to follow-up as of this study; both had progressed well postoperatively and had been fitted with temporary prosthetic devices. The third patient had difficulty ambulating because of the weight of her prosthesis and was using a wheelchair at the time of her last visit. One patient died due to comorbid medical conditions approximately 2 years after the Syme's amputation.

Discussion

Complete disarticulation or amputation of the foot is not a pleasant thought for either patients or physicians, although at times it is desirable, necessary, and readily accepted by patients who have been plagued with a dysfunctional foot for a prolonged period. Patients with severe deformity not amenable to surgical correction; severe intractable chronic pain syndromes; severe recurrent or chronic ulcerations, especially ulcers associated with underlying osteomyelitis; and malignancy or severe crush injuries are often best served by an amputation procedure.

Syme's procedure has been shown to an effective alternative to below-knee amputation and is greatly underused by orthopedic, vascular, and podiatric surgeons. It is hoped that this article will stimulate and encourage colleagues to consider this approach when amputation has been determined to be the best approach for any given patient. The procedure consistently produces a functional limb, with maximal length preservation, which when fitted with a well-designed and constructed prosthesis results in a near-normal gait pattern and cadence with minimal increased energy expenditure. Compared with more traditional amputations, including below-knee amputation and midtarsal joint amputation, Syme's amputation is more energy efficient.

The senior author came to appreciate this procedure by accident when at the prodding of senior podiatric residents was convinced that a Syme's amputation was clearly preferred over a below-knee amputation, which had been advised by several other surgeon specialists for a patient after a severe crush injury at a construction site. The 25-year-old, otherwise healthy man, given the alternatives, was advised of the rationale and given a realistic picture of what could be attained with this approach. Because his foot already had undergone a guillotine amputation at the midtarsal joint with no soft tissue flap preservation or coverage, his options were severely limited. He underwent a Syme's amputation and made a rapid recovery. Today, 5 years later, he continues to be fully ambulatory with no obvious or significant gait alterations. He has no obvious limp. When dressed with full-length slacks one would not be able to select him out from any other person in an everyday crowd of people walking about. Since that time, the author has continued to recommend and perform this procedure for a variety of pathologies as reviewed earlier in this article with favorable outcomes.

There are many subtle but nonetheless important considerations when contemplating this procedure. A good understanding and realistic expectations by the patient lie at the heart of success with this procedure. A straightforward, compassionate, and empathetic face-to-face dialogue is helpful in alleviating fears and doubts; the patient's significant other or family members should be encouraged to participate in the discussion and provide additional mental, physical, and emotional support. There may be psychological issues with female patients with regard to the overall penile shape and appearance of the limb after amputation of the foot. For some women, this appearance may preclude them from undergoing a Syme's amputation in lieu of a below-knee amputation. Although this comment has been made to the senior author on more than one occasion, no female patient selected a below-knee amputation over a Syme's amputation to date.

The authors always recommend that patients meet with a highly experienced orthotist, prosthetist, or pedorthist to learn more about the process of the temporary and later permanent prosthetic device, including the opportunity to see and touch an actual device; this is an area of likely failure by many surgeons resulting in high levels of frustration for the patient and surgeon. We cannot overemphasize the importance of the surgeon in identifying a highly skilled, knowledgeable, and, more importantly, experienced professional to design, fabricate, and fit the prosthesis. The successful outcome depends on these interrelationships. Without them, the patient may never be ambulatory again. Finally, the authors also offer patients the opportunity to talk with others who have undergone the same procedure to increase further their comfort level with their decision to have the foot amputated.

The preoperative evaluation and assessment also is important to a successful outcome. In addition to confirmation of a good heel pad, which serves as the weight-bearing load area postoperatively, the arterial circulation at the level of the ankle joint must be sufficient to support wound healing. As discussed earlier, numerous noninvasive vascular study techniques have been shown to be reliable predictors of success and failure. We encourage the use of these parameters to predict the likelihood of complication. The patient's nutritional status also should be investigated. Wound complications are increased significantly in patients who have malnutrition, a problem readily rectified with minimal effort and consultation. Comorbidities should be assessed carefully to ensure the best possible overall health status before surgery; diabetic patients should have optimal blood glucose levels, not only during the surgery, but also throughout the perioperative period to minimize complications. Antibiotic prophylaxis is recommended for the first 24 hours given the risk of the procedure and the fact that many patients undergoing this procedure already will have suffered from chronic soft tissue and bone infections. Prophylaxis for thromboembolic phenomenon, such as deep vein thrombophlebitis or pulmonary embolism, also should be considered; when significant risk factors are identified, pharmacologic prophylaxis with a low-molecular-weight heparin or warfarin (Coumadin) is prescribed. Mechanical prophylaxis also is used during surgery on the contralateral extremity.

The surgical procedure itself is not overly difficult. A working knowledge of the entire anatomy about the foot and ankle greatly facilitates efficient disarticulation of the foot. Emphasis is placed on carefully planned incisions to ensure sufficient plantar flap coverage of the distal stump and minimal tension on the wound edges. The individual nerves should be identified and severed as far proximal as possible to encourage retraction and, it is hoped, minimize stump neuroma formation. The osseous resection of the malleoli should be confirmed intraoperatively with C-arm fluoroscopy or conventional radiographs because the contour and shape of the stump greatly affect the quality and fit of the prosthesis; a wide distal stump is likely to be problematic with prosthesis fitting. The distal articular surface of the tibia can be left intact or resected, depending on the preference of the surgeon. If a tourniquet is employed for hemostasis, it should be released before closure. Meticulous technique and close attention to closure of the skin help to minimize postoperative wound complications, which are common in the authors' experience. Finally, the application of a multilayered compression bandage is effective in minimizing postoperative edema and facilitates shrinkage of the stump over 4 to 6 weeks.

References

[1] Letts M. Surgical cases and amputations: Amputation at the ankle- joint. Clin Orthop 1990;256: 3–6.
[2] Harris RI. Syme's amputation: The technical details essential for success. J Bone Joint Surg Br 1956;38-B(3):614–32.

[3] Wagner FW. A classification and treatment program for diabetic, neurotrophic and dysvascular foot problems. Instructional Course Lectures, The American Academy of Orthopaedic Surgeons, vol. 28. Mosby. p. 143–65.

[4] Catterall RC. Syme's amputation by Joseph Lister after sixty-six years. J Bone Joint Surg Br 1967;49-B(1):144.

[5] Ratliff AHC. Syme's amputation: Result after forty-four years. J Bone Joint Surg Br 1967; 49-B(1):142–3.

[6] Baker GCW, Stableforth PG. Syme's amputation: A review of sixty-seven cases. J Bone Joint Surg Br 1969;51-B(3):482–7.

[7] Lin-Chan S, Nielsen DH. Physiological Responses to multiple speed treadmill walking for Syme vs transtibial amputation – a case report. Disabil Rehabil 2003;25(23):1333–8.

[8] Satterfield K. Amputation Considerations and Energy Expenditures in the Diabetic Patient. Clinics in Podiatric Medicine and Surgery 2003;20:793–801.

[9] Bowker JH, San Giovanni TP. Amputation and disarticulations, ch. 17. In: Myerson MS, editor. Foot and Ankle Disorders, vol. 2. Philadelphia: W.B. Saunders; 2000. p. 466–98.

[10] Bowker JH, San Giovanni TP. Minor and major lower limb amputations in persons with diabetes mellitus, ch. 28. In: Bowker JH, Pfeifer MA, editors. Levin and O'Neal's The Diabetic Foot. 6th ed. St. Louis: Mosby; 2001. p. 627–32.

[11] Malone JW. Lower extremity amputation, ch. 44. In: Moore WS, editor. Vascular Surgery: A Comprehensive Review. 4th ed. Philadelphia: W.B. Saunders; 1993. p. 822–4.

[12] Dickhaut SC, DeLee JC, Page CP. Nutrional status: Importance in predicting wound-healing after amputation. J Bone Joint Surg Am 1984;66-A(1):71–5.

[13] Pinzur MS, Sage R, Stuck R, et al. Transcutaneous oxygen as a predictor of wound healing in amputations of the foot and ankle. Foot Ankle Int 1992;13(5):271–2.

[14] Pinzur MS, Stuck R, Sage R, et al. Transcutaneous oxygen tension in the dysvacular foot with infection. Foot Ankle Int 1993;14(5):254–6.

[15] Biomechanical Markers of Nutritional Status: Malnutrition in Hospitalized Patients. Regional Laboratory Alliance Newsletter 1998;13(7).

[16] Pagano KD. Protein Components Test. Mosby's Manual of Diagnostic and Laboratory Tests. St. Louis: Mosby, Inc.; 1998.

[17] Basu HN, Liepa GU. Arginine: A Clinical Perspective. Nutr Clin Practice 2002;17:218–25.

[18] Witte MB, Banbal A. Role of Nitric Oxide in Wound Repair. Am J Surg 2002;183:406–12.

[19] Mayfield JA, Reiber GE, Sanders LJ, et al. Preventive Foot Care in People with Diabetes. Diabetes Care 2002;20(12):2161–77.

[20] Pinzur M. Syme Ankle Disarticulation in Diabetic Dysvascular Disease and Trauma. Techniques in Foot and Ankle Surgery 2004;3(1):15–22.

[21] Spittler AW, Brennan JJ, Payne JW. Syme amputation performed in two stages. J Bone Joint Surg Am 1954;36-A:37.

[22] Pinzur MS, Morrison C, Sage R, Stuck R, et al. Syme's two-stage amputation in insulin-requiring diabetics with gangrene of the forefoot. Foot Ankle Int 1991;11(6):394–6.

[23] Pinzur MS, Smith D, Osterman H. Syme ankle disarticulation in peripheral vascular disease and diabetic foot infection: The one-stage versus the two-stage procedure. Foot Ankle Int 1995;16(3):124–7.

[24] Jahss MH, Michelson JD, Desai P, et al. Investigations into the fat pads of the sole of the foot: Anatomy and Histology. Foot Ankle Int 1992;13(5):233–42.

[25] Robinson KP. Disarticulation at the ankle using an anterior flap. J Bone Joint Surg Br 1999; 81-B:617–20.

[26] Smith DG, Sangeorzan BJ, Hansen ST, et al. Achilles tendon tenodesis to prevent heel pad migration in the Syme's amputation. Foot Ankle Int 1994;15(1):14–7.

[27] Pinzur MS. Restoration of walking ability with Syme's ankle disarticulation. Clin Orthop 1999; 361:71–5.

[28] Cottrell-Ikerd V, Ikerd F, Jenkins DW. The Syme's amputation: A correlation of surgical technique and prosthetic management with a historical perspective. J Foot Ankle Surg 1994;33(4): 335–64.

[29] Radcliffe CW. The biomechanics of the Syme prosthesis. Artif Limbs 1961;6:76–85.
[30] The Canadian Association of Prosthetist and Orthotists. Socket designs for the Syme's amputee, ch. 3.6. In: Weber D, editor. Clinical Aspects of Lower Extremity Prosthetics. Oakville, Ontario: Elgan Enterprises; 1991. p. 169–74.
[31] Prosthetic Manual. ch. 18. Chicago, IL: Northwestern University Medical School Prosthetic-Orthotic Center; 1993. p. 227A–227H.
[32] Sarmiento A. A modified surgical-prosthetic approach to the Syme's amputation: a follow-up report. Clin Orthop 1972;85:11–5.
[33] Waters RL, Perry J, Antonelli D, et al. Energy cost of walking amputees: the influence of level of amputation. J Bone Joint Surg Am 1976;58-A:43–6.
[34] Sinclair WF. Below the knee and Syme's amputation prostheses. Orthop Clin North Am 1972;3: 349–57.
[35] Wagner FW. Amputations of the foot and ankle: Current status. Clin Orthop 1977;122:62–9.
[36] Pinzur MS. Amputation level selection in the diabetic foot. Clin Orthop 1993;296:68–70.
[37] Pinzur MS, Wolf B, Havey RM. Walking pattern of midfoot and ankle disarticulation amputees. Foot Ankle Int 1997;18(10):635–8.
[38] Pinzur MS, Stuck RM, et al. Syme ankle disarticulation in patients with diabetes. JBJS 2003; 85-A(9):1667–72.

ELSEVIER
SAUNDERS

Clin Podiatr Med Surg
22 (2005) 429–446

CLINICS IN
PODIATRIC
MEDICINE AND
SURGERY

When Is a More Proximal Amputation Needed?

Robert W. Zickler, MD[a,b,]*, Frank T. Padberg, Jr, MD[a,b],
Brajesh K. Lal, MD[a], Peter J. Pappas, MD[a]

[a]*Division of Vascular Surgery, New Jersey Medical School,
University of Medicine and Dentistry of New Jersey, PO Box 1709, Newark, NJ 07101, USA*
[b]*Section of Vascular Surgery, Veterans Affairs New Jersey Health Care Systems, 385 Tremont Avenue,
East Orange, NJ 07019, USA*

Amputation may be the most appropriate therapy for an ischemic or infected limb. In the United States, 60,000 to 120,000 amputations are performed annually, with greater than 90% of them for gangrene resulting from ischemia or infection [1,2]. Indications for amputation include: (1) gangrene, nonhealing ulcers, refractory infection, and rest pain caused by nonreconstructable arterial disease, (2) irreversible tissue damage from ischemia, and (3) fulminant foot infections in diabetics. The level at which to amputate is often difficult to determine, however. Numerous studies over the past two decades have reported early mortality from a major amputation and for surgical revision as high as 20% or more [3–11].

The goals in selecting an amputation site are: (1) removal of nonsalvageable tissue, (2) relief of pain, (3) achievement of primary healing, and (4) preservation of as much limb length as possible [12,13]. With the number of amputations steadily increasing, especially in diabetic patients, meeting these goals is particularly important. They help optimize the rehabilitation potential of the patient and avoid the risks of a second surgical procedure [14,15].

Maintaining maximal limb length increases the success of rehabilitation [16]. For example, compared with normal walking in a nonamputee, there is almost no increase in energy expenditure for a toe amputation and the potential for rehabilitation should be 100%. Even an ankle-level amputation, such as a Syme or Pirogoff, requires no more than a 10% increase in energy consumption and

* Corresponding author. Veterans Affairs Medical Center, 385 Tremont Avenue, East Orange, NJ 07019.

E-mail address: robert.zickler@med.va.gov (R.W. Zickler).

0891-8422/05/$ – see front matter © 2005 Elsevier Inc. All rights reserved.
doi:10.1016/j.cpm.2005.03.002   *podiatric.theclinics.com*

most patients resume normal daily and work-related activities [1]. The energy expenditure for ambulating with a unilateral below-knee amputation is increased 10% to 40%. Approximately 70% of these patients will attain bipedal gait. Patients with a unilateral above-knee amputation have a 50% to 57% increase in energy expenditure with only 10% to 30% walking again [17–19].

The more distal the amputation, however, the greater the risk for wound breakdown leading to a more proximal amputation [3,20]. Despite improvement in limb salvage rates in patients with vascular insufficiency resulting from technical advances in lower-extremity revascularization, the number of amputations performed yearly has not decreased [21]. This is a result of the continuous increase in the mean age of the population and the greater prevalence of amputations in older patients [22–24]. Infectious complications and vascular compromise caused by diabetes mellitus account for most lower-extremity amputations [25,26]. Ten to fifteen percent of diabetic patients will require a major or minor amputation [27]. Approximately half of these amputations are performed at the level of the foot [28]. Fifteen to thirty-five percent of diabetics with a lower-extremity amputation will require an amputation on the opposite leg within 5 years [29,30].

Between 10% and 50% of amputations will require a revision of the surgical site [4,12,31,32]. This may be a result of inappropriate selection of the initial amputation site [14]. In many cases, one of two approaches has been used to select the level of amputation. The first is to perform the most distal amputation and progressively revise to a higher level until healing ultimately occurs. This places the patient at risk from multiple anesthetics and multiple surgical procedures. The other approach is to select an amputation site with sufficient blood flow to ensure healing. This is often at a higher level than necessary and compromises the patient's rehabilitation potential. Neither of these methods is satisfactory.

The microcirculation and oxygenation of the tissue surrounding an area are the most important factors for wound healing [27]. Clinical evaluation is not a reliable predictor of successful healing of an amputation level when used alone [12,31–33]. The best prediction of wound healing is based on the clinical assessment of an experienced surgeon aided by one of several ancillary tests [1]. A diagnostic test that could determine accurately the ability of an amputation to heal would reduce cost and patient suffrage by eliminating long, unsuccessful attempts at conservative management. It also could prevent amputations that are more proximal than necessary, reducing a patient's chance for rehabilitation.

Although clinical judgment remains the primary method used to determine the level of amputation [34,35], multiple diagnostic tests can help guide the surgeon, including segmental systolic blood pressure measurements, fluorescein dye measurements, laser Doppler flowmetry, skin perfusion pressures, isotope measurement of skin blood flow, transcutaneous oxygen tension, and transcutaneous carbon dioxide tension [36]. These studies supply objective criteria to help determine the most optimal level of amputation. None is ideal, however, and they must be tailored to the individual's need. In addition, the anatomic considerations and multiple perioperative issues that affect the selection of an amputation site must be addressed.

Objective considerations in determining amputation level

Clinical judgment

Physical findings used to clinically select an amputation level include skin condition at the presumed amputation site, hair over the toes, thickened toenails, pallor with foot elevation, temperature, color, presence or absence of pulses, vascularity of the muscle and skin, presence of dependent ischemic rubor, and gangrene at the proposed level of amputation (Box 1). Clinical judgment used alone will predict successful healing in approximately 90% of above-knee amputations and 80% of below-knee amputations [37–39].

Prediction of successful healing for amputations below the ankle is only 40% when relying on clinical judgment alone [40]. The presence of gangrene and dependent rubor at the proposed amputation site are the most reliable predictors of failure. Both are signs of severe ischemia. Their absence does not ensure success, however [36]. Amputations performed immediately below the most distal palpable pulse have excellent healing potential. The absence of a pulse does not mean the wound is doomed to failure, however [41–43]. Similarly, subjective assessment of skin condition, temperature, color, and vascularity also may lead to a suboptimal selection of amputation level. Although clinical judgment alone is insufficient, the value of an experienced surgeon should not be underemphasized. The addition of objective studies can improve the chances of healing at the most distal level of amputation and supplement clinical judgment, although they cannot replace it (Box 2) [44].

Box 1. Clinical evaluation in determining amputation level

Skin condition
Distribution of hair
Thickening of toenails
Skin temperature
Skin color
Pulses
Pallor with elevation
Dependent rubor
Gangrene
Intraoperative vascularity

Box 2. Diagnostic tests in determining amputation level

Segmental systolic blood pressure measurements
Pulse volume recordings
Transcutaneous oxygen tension (TcPO$_2$)
Fluorescein dye
Laser Doppler flowmetry
Skin perfusion pressures
Skin blood flow
Skin temperature

Segmental systolic blood pressure measurements

Hemodynamic parameters such as Doppler segmental pressures and ankle/brachial indices give useful information on the degree of arterial insufficiency [45]. These parameters evaluate the macrocirculation, which indirectly reflects the microcirculation [46,47]. Systolic pressures and ankle/brachial indices are inexpensive and easy to perform, but their accuracy varies [48]. These methods, however, can aid in the selection of an amputation site, particularly at the above-knee or below-knee level [49]. They are far less reliable at the level of the foot [48,50,51]. Also, definitive values used to predict successful healing of an amputation site vary widely [45].

The shortcoming of these techniques is that they do not measure perfusion at the level of the skin, where critical limb ischemia occurs [52]. The value of Doppler systolic pressures also is limited in noncompressible calcified vessels [27,33,53,54]. This condition is particularly common in diabetic patients, leading to falsely elevated pressures and inaccurate information [55–57]. These patients form a significant percentage of those requiring amputation [12,15]. Toe systolic blood pressures are a more reliable index in this subset of patients because the digital arteries are less affected by medial calcification. Toe pressures less than 30 mm Hg are an indicator of poor wound healing [54]. Toe pressures cannot be measured, however, if there is extensive ulceration or gangrene, if the toes are thickly callused, or if the toes are absent as a result of prior amputations [58].

Pulse volume recordings

Microcirculatory changes resulting from peripheral arterial disease decrease tissue perfusion and are responsible for critical ischemia [59]. Pulse volume recordings reflect the state of blood flow in the arterial system [60]. The amplitude of the pulse wave is proportional to the quantity of blood flow at that site and can be used as an indicator of distal perfusion [60,61]. Pulse volume recordings from the toes can provide objective data as to the healing potential of an amputation in the foot. They also have been recommended for evaluation of the circulation in diabetics because they are prone to medial calcification [47]. Pulse waves from the toes can be obtained readily with the use of photoplethysmography [62]. Measurements are taken with the patient at rest. A uniform temperature is obtained with a heating blanket to eliminate the effects of temperature [62,63]. Pulse waves are recorded from the plantar aspect of the toes with their amplitude measured in millimeters [62]. Low pulse volume recordings are an indicator of tissue ischemia and predict wound-healing failure [60]. Wave amplitude in combination with Doppler systolic pressures help predict better the most appropriate level of amputation. There is no definitive pulse wave amplitude below which tissue viability cannot be supported, however. Pulse waves follow a range, with poorer prognosis with lower amplitude waveforms and better prognosis with higher amplitude waveforms [62]. Therefore, pulse waves can help guide therapy but can only predict outcome.

Transcutaneous oxygen tension (TcPO$_2$)

Multiple studies have demonstrated the diagnostic advantages of TcPO$_2$ measurements in evaluation of the arterial supply to the lower extremities [33,57, 64–66]. TcPO$_2$ can help guide therapy because it can predict reliably the presence of significant arterial compromise [45,64]. TcPO$_2$ reflects the local macro- and microcirculation. It is influenced by central factors, such as arterial oxygen content, and local factors, such as tissue perfusion and oxygen consumption [27,57,67,68]. A threshold of cutaneous blood flow is necessary to heal an amputation suture line successfully. TcPO$_2$ measurements correlate with cutaneous oxygen content, which assesses cutaneous blood flow [55,69]. This makes TcPO$_2$ a useful parameter for the selection of the most distal amputation site [33,70–73]. The reliability of TcPO$_2$ measurements is similar in diabetic and nondiabetic patients [74,75]. It is not affected by medial calcific sclerosis, which is prevalent in the diabetic population. This allows for a more universal application in almost all patients who require an amputation [33].

The technique needs to be performed in a uniform manner to get reliable and reproducible results [76]. Patients are placed in a supine position for 15 to 20 minutes to achieve a steady state while breathing room air. The room temperature is maintained between 24 and 26°C. The sensor is heated to 44 or 45°C to increase the permeability of the skin to oxygen molecules [27,33,45]. Measurements are taken at the level of the proposed amputation site [77]. The test takes approximately 30 minutes to 1 hour to perform [58].

As with other diagnostic tools, there is a range of values with the lower the measurement, the lower the probability of healing [10,72,78,79]. The wide range of TcPO$_2$ values reported by different investigators as the cutoff for critical ischemia is a major shortcoming of this test [12,33,45]. Amputation sites with a TcPO$_2$ value greater than 30 mm Hg have a high likelihood of healing [45,57], whereas values less than 20 mm Hg are more likely to fail [36]. There is no threshold value below which an amputation site definitely will fail to heal. Although unlikely, a wound still might heal with a TcPO$_2$ of 0 mm Hg [12,77,80].

By combining the $TcPO_2$ value with a patient's clinical status, the amputation level can be selected better. For example, the risk for a second surgery is lower in a young and otherwise healthy diabetic patient and it may be worth performing an amputation at a level where the $TcPO_2$ is lower. Although the rate of stump failure may be higher, it maximizes the patient's chance of rehabilitation. In contrast, in an elderly patient with multiple medical problems and high anesthetic risk, a higher $TcPO_2$ with a greater chance of healing the amputation site might be more appropriate [12].

Fluorescein dye

Objective quantification of fluorescein in the skin by fiber-optic perfusion fluorometry seems to be reliable in selecting amputation level [81–83]. After intravenous administration of fluorescein dye, the fluorescein diffuses into the extracellular fluid. The amount of fluorescein in the tissue is directly proportional to the perfusion of the tissue [84]. By exposing the interstitial fluorescein to blue light, a bright green fluorescence is produced that can be quantified. A dual channel fluorometer is used. One channel transmits the blue light and the other channel measures the amount of fluorescence [85]. The higher the numerical value obtained by the fluorometer, the greater the blood flow at the site and the greater the likelihood of wound healing.

There are several advantages to this technique. First, multiple measurements can be obtained at different levels of the limb, as well as circumferentially around the proposed amputation site. Second, fluorometry is not affected by diabetes mellitus and medial arterial calcification [81]. In addition, the technique is as reliable for amputations in the foot as it is for amputations of the leg. Fiber-optic fluorometry has a greater accuracy in predicting the appropriate level of amputation than clinical judgment alone [81,83]. The major shortcoming of this test is that it is not reliable in the presence of cellulitis, inflammation, or edema [83,86]. Extravasation of fluorescein through the endothelium of the capillary bed at these sites gives unreliable readings. Because inflammation often accompanies gangrene or impending tissue loss, this technique has not gained widespread use [36].

Laser Doppler flowmetry

Laser Doppler flowmetry is based on the principle of the Doppler effect. A laser beam is generated by the device and directed at the skin surface. The light is scattered by the objects in its path. Moving objects such as red blood cells cause a frequency shift in the backscatter. The degree of shift is proportional to the velocity of the moving object. Static structures such as the skin do not cause a frequency shift. The return signal is recorded and processed by the probe's photodetector. A numerical value is obtained that is directly proportional to the blood flow in the microcirculation. The depth of penetration of the light beam is limited to approximately 1 mm, preventing interference from deeper vessels. This allows for evaluation of the skin microcirculation and skin blood flow.

Laser Doppler flow measurements do not correlate to cutaneous blood flow in nonheated skin. If the skin is not heated, the values fall in the same general range for patients with significant arterial disease as those without [87,88]. By heating the skin beneath the laser probe, a hyperemic response is elicited. This hyperemic response is delayed markedly and diminished in patients with significant arterial insufficiency [89]. By heating the skin, the laser Doppler measurements correlate in a linear fashion with skin perfusion and allow for a more accurate selection of amputation level. Laser Doppler flowmetry measurements can be obtained reliably at all levels of proposed amputation from above-knee to the toes.

Skin perfusion pressures

Skin perfusion pressure is defined as the minimal amount of external compression needed to stop microcirculatory blood flow in the skin. It provides an objective measurement of limb ischemia and can be used to evaluate the healing potential of proposed amputation sites [90,91]. It is a physiologic test that is not affected by medial calcific sclerosis, allowing its use in nearly all patients [58]. Skin perfusion pressures also can be obtained anywhere on the limb where viable tissue is present. Several methods for obtaining skin perfusion pressures have been described including laser Doppler, photoplethysmography, and isotope washout [41,58,92]. The simplest method for obtaining skin perfusion pressures is with a laser Doppler. The device consists of a laser Doppler probe inside a blood pressure cuff modified with a transparent plastic window. The laser Doppler is directed through the window and onto the patient's skin. The cuff is inflated to a suprasystolic level and gradually allowed to deflate. The pressure at which microcirculatory skin blood flow returns is the skin perfusion pressure [58]. Warming the skin may increase the reliability of the test [93]. Average testing is approximately 15 minutes for each site [91]. Photoelectric plethysmography uses a similar technique as laser Doppler.

Another method used to obtain skin perfusion pressures is the isotope washout technique. In this technique, a radioactive isotope such as ^{131}I-antipyrine or ^{99m}pertechnate is injected intradermally at the proposed site of amputation. A scintillation counter is used to monitor the level of the isotope. A blood pressure cuff is placed over the injection site and inflated until clearance of the isotope stops. The pressure at which this occurs is recorded as the skin perfusion pressure [53]. The threshold value for skin perfusion pressure seems to be between 20 and 30 mm Hg. Pressures above this level predict reliable healing, whereas pressures below this level predict failure of healing [41,58,91,94]. One disadvantage of skin perfusion pressures is that they are not as accurate with minor amputations as they are with major amputations [91].

Laser Doppler and photoelectric plethysmography have several advantages over the isotope washout technique for determining skin perfusion pressures. First, they can be repeated quickly multiple times to verify the results. The devices are also portable, enabling the test to be performed at the bedside. In addition, radioisotopes are not necessary, eliminating the complexity and expense of the equipment, the need for specialized technicians, and discomfort to the patient [33,91].

Skin blood flow

Adequate skin blood flow is essential for wound healing. By measuring skin blood flow with radioactive tracers, an accurate predictor of amputation healing at multiple levels can be obtained [95]. Much of the literature studying skin blood flow uses [133]xenon. Because this agent is no longer commercially available, however, other isotopes such as iodine 125 iodoantipyrine have been used. The technique involves an intradermal injection [95] or epicutaneous application [96] of the radioactive gas. With the epicutaneous method, the agent diffuses into the skin but is unable to diffuse back out [97]. Whether injected or allowed to diffuse into the skin, the radionucleotide is cleared by the capillaries of the dermis. A conventional gamma camera is used to measure the amount of agent present. The rate of removal of the isotope is proportional to the blood flow at that site. The more rapidly the tracer is removed, the greater the blood flow, which is measured in mL/100 g of tissue/min. The major drawback of this technique has been the difficulty in obtaining standardized values from one institution to another. The values range from 1 mL/100 g of tissue/min [95] to 2.4 mL/100 g of tissue/min [98] as the lowest blood flow consistent with healing of an amputation site. Others have recommended values between these [96,99]. Despite this shortcoming, experienced investigators have shown skin blood flow to be accurate in predicting primary healing of amputations with 83% healing at the toe level, 93% healing at the below-knee level, and 100% healing at the above-knee level [100,101].

Skin temperature

Although subjective evaluation of skin temperature by tactile examination does not correlate well with amputation healing [102], objective thermometry may [103,104]. Skin temperature is related directly to skin blood flow [105]. The use of cutaneous temperature in predicting wound healing at a selected level of amputation may be helpful. If the skin temperature is greater than 32°C at the amputation site, the chance of healing is greater than 94%. Also, if the difference in temperature between the proposed amputation site and the ambient temperature is greater than 5°C, primary healing will occur in greater than 92% [80,106]. Thermometry is a noninvasive, inexpensive, and simple test to assess skin blood flow objectively. The major shortcoming of this technique is the lack of a uniform temperature in the various studies below which primary healing will not occur. Because other techniques for evaluating amputation sites are more applicable, little research in this field has been performed in recent years.

Anatomic considerations in determining amputation level

Box 3 lists anatomic considerations in determining amputation level.

Toe and ray amputations

A toe amputation is indicated for infection or gangrene localized to the distal or middle phalanx. If the disease process extends to the metatarsophalangeal region, a ray amputation is the appropriate treatment. Contraindications to a toe or ray amputation include arterial insufficiency and dependent rubor at the proposed level of amputation, and evidence of proximal infection. Physical examination can help predict successful healing. If palpable pedal pulses are present, there is a 98% chance of healing [107]. Empirical section in the absence of palpable pedal pulses yields only a 75% chance of successful healing [108]. Photoplethysmographic transmetatarsal or toe pressures greater than 20 mm Hg or Doppler ankle pressure greater than 35 mm Hg predict successful healing in 100% and 96%, respectively [109,110]. Other techniques are less reliable in predicting successful healing [36].

Transmetatarsal and midfoot amputations

A transmetatarsal amputation is indicated for infection or gangrene involving several toes but not extending much past the metatarsophalangeal crease. Arterial

---

Box 3. Anatomic considerations in determining amputation level

Toe and ray amputation
   Pedal pulses
   Photoplethysmographic skin perfusion pressures
   Doppler pressures
Transmetatarsal amputations
   $TcPO_2$
   Skin blood flow
   Fluorescein dye measurements
Midfoot and ankle-level amputations
   Doppler pressures
   Skin blood flow
   Fluorescein dye measurements

(*Data from* Durham JR. Lower extremity amputation levels: indications, determining the appropriate level, technique, and prognosis. In: Rutherford RB, editor. Vascular Surgery. 5th edition. Philadelphia: WB Saunders; 2000. p. 2185–213.)

insufficiency and dependent rubor at the proposed level of amputation or evidence of proximal infection preclude a transmetatarsal amputation. If a plantar space infection is present or the plantar skin is compromised, a more proximal amputation must be performed. Several methods are accurate in predicting successful healing at the transmetatarsal level. TcPO$_2$ level of 20 mm Hg predicts successful healing in only 50% of amputations, whereas a TcPO$_2$ of 40 mm Hg predicts a 90% chance of healing [45]. Transcutaneous carbon dioxide (TcPO$_2$) level may also be effective in predicting healing [100]. There are less data available on TcPO$_2$ assays, however, and further investigation is required.

Skin blood flow determination with xenon or iodine 125 iodoantipyrine greater than 2.6 mL/100 g tissue/min will yield a 92% successful healing rate [100]. Fiber-optic perfusion fluorometry with a dye fluorescence index of greater than 44 predicts a 90% likelihood of wound healing [83]. If the above tests are not available, systolic blood pressure measurements may provide useful information. A Doppler ankle pressure greater than 60 or 70 mm Hg suggests that 75% of transmetatarsal amputations will heal [50,111,112], whereas below 40 mm Hg predicts failure [113]. Photoplethysmographic toe pressures greater than 55 mm Hg predict reliable healing of a transmetatarsal amputation and below 55 mm Hg predict failure [54]. Lastly, pulse volume recordings with normal amplitude and waveform at the level of amputation provide a reliable index of successful healing [36].

Midfoot amputations such as those of Chopart and Lisfranc are indicated if infection or gangrene precludes a transmetatarsal amputation. If arterial insufficiency is present at the proposed level of amputation, efforts should be made to revascularize the foot or the wound will fail to heal. A Doppler ankle pressure of greater than 30 mm Hg is the most reliable predictor of healing of midfoot amputations. An ankle pressure less than 30 mm Hg predicts failure [114,115]. TcPO$_2$ values are not useful predictors of healing in midfoot amputations. They are inaccurate over the thick plantar skin upon which these amputations are based.

Ankle-level amputations

An ankle-level amputation such as a Pirogoff or Syme is indicated for a distal forefoot infection that involves the plantar skin or fascia. Transmetatarsal and midfoot amputations are contraindicated in this situation because they require healthy plantar skin distally. This is not required in an ankle-level amputation. Contraindications to an ankle-level amputation include ischemia, dependent rubor, neuropathy, and any abnormality of the heel such as ulceration, gangrene, or infection. Arterial insufficiency at the proposed amputation site precludes an ankle-level amputation because healing of the skin flap demands a good blood supply from the posterior tibial artery. If ischemia is present at the proposed level of amputation, efforts should be made to revascularize the tissue. The same objective studies used to predict healing in forefoot amputations are helpful in patients being considered for ankle-level amputations [36].

Perioperative issues affecting amputation level

Box 4 lists perioperative issues affecting amputation level.

Preoperative Issues

Multiple preoperative issues may need to be addressed when determining the level of amputation. Osteomyelitis requires preoperative antibiotic therapy, if possible, to eradicate the bony infection. If this is unsuccessful, the amputation must be performed proximal to the infection. If the amputation is done near the site of osteomyelitis, it has been suggested that a specimen from the margin of the transected bone be sent for culture [116]. If the culture comes back positive and the site fails to heal, a revision will need to be performed in a noninfected site.

Antibiotic therapy also needs to be initiated for soft tissue infections surrounding a proposed amputation site. A staged procedure such as an open amputation may be needed to prevent the spread of infection. Once the infection has

---

Box 4. Perioperative issues affecting amputation level

Preoperative
    Osteomyelitis
    Soft tissue infection
    Neuropathy
    Diabetes mellitus
    Renal insufficiency
    Venous hypertension
    Prior surgery at site
    Smoking
Intraoperative
    Vascularity
    Muscle contractility
    Suture material
    Surgical technique
    Hemostasis
Postoperative
    Infection
    Hematoma
    Ischemia
    Trauma to site
    Callus formation
    Neuroma formation
    Bone spur formation
    Scar tissue

resolved after the open procedure, revision to a formal amputation is performed. This allows for the most conservative amputation possible.

Patients with peripheral neuropathies also require special consideration. Diminished sensation places these patients at risk for developing plantar ulcers. With early diagnosis, the ulcers can be treated with local wound care and pressure relief. If an amputation at any level in the foot is considered it should be performed proximal to the level of neuropathy if possible, however, because recurrent ulceration is common [116].

Several medical conditions also can compromise the skin or soft tissue flaps of an amputation. Diabetes mellitus and renal failure affect the microcirculation and lead to vascular insufficiency, especially of the skin. Venous hypertension resulting from an existing or previous deep venous thrombosis (DVT) also can affect healing at the amputation site. DVT occurs from 5% to 40% in patients undergoing amputation [116,117]. The resulting edema can cause separation of the wound edges and compromise the surgical site. Compression may aid the healing process in these cases, but is contraindicated if the amputation was the result of arterial insufficiency. In addition, scars from prior incisions may affect the surgical field adversely. The skin between the old incision and the new one is particularly vulnerable. To prevent this, the old scar should be excised or at least incorporated into the new incision. Lastly, smokers are twice as likely as nonsmokers for amputation site infection and the need for a more proximal re-amputation. Smokers need to stop smoking for at least 1 week before surgery to diminish the vasoconstrictive effects of nicotine [118].

Intraoperative issues

Several intraoperative factors may affect healing potential. If the skin does not bleed or the muscle does not contract with stimulation at the proposed level, a more proximal amputation is necessary. Foreign material such as bone wax and silk sutures need to be avoided. The tissues should be handled gently and the skin edges avoided. The skin should not be manipulated with surgical instruments. If necessary, the subcutaneous tissue should be picked up and not the skin. Any minor trauma can cause a focal necrosis and lead to healing failure. Upon closure of the wound, the skin edges should be approximated gently. Excessive tension can lead to vascular compromise and necrosis of the skin edges. In addition, the wound needs to be hemostatic before closure because hematoma formation can compromise healing.

Postoperative issues

Various postoperative complications also can lead to poor wound healing at the amputation site. Infection can prevent healing and often requires revision to a more proximal level. Amputation site infections range from 12% to 28% depending on the reason for the amputation [119,120]. Patients undergoing amputation secondary to infection should receive antibiotic coverage specific for the causative agent as determined by culture. Patients undergoing amputation for noninfectious reasons need to receive perioperative prophylactic antibiotics. Hematoma in the surgical field also must be avoided because of the high correlation of hematoma and infection [116]. Ischemia can lead to ulceration or healing failure of the amputation, necessitating revision to a higher level. Appropriate vascular reconstruction performed before amputation or for a failing surgical site may help lower the level of amputation or salvage a compromised site. Precautions also must be taken to prevent inadvertent trauma by the patient to the surgical field. Protective dressings and footwear and patient education are mandatory to protect the amputation site. If the incision separates as a result of trauma, revision to a higher level is often necessary.

Multiple issues may lead to late complications and failure of a well-healed amputation. Callus formation is common over bony prominences. If a bony prominence exists at the amputation site, a callus can cause pain or erosion of the soft tissue. Pain also can result from neuroma formation within the surgical field. Transecting the nerve deep in the muscle is the best way to minimize its occurrence. In addition, a bone spur can form around the circumference of the transected bone. It can lead to pain, callus formation, or pressure necrosis of the soft tissue. Bone spur formation can be minimized by limiting the amount of periosteal stripping during the procedure. Lastly, scar tissue is less resistant to shear stresses and will break down easier than normal tissue. Careful preoperative planning is necessary to prevent incisions and scar tissue on weight-bearing surfaces.

Summary

Selecting the appropriate level is crucial when performing an amputation. The goals of surgery are to maintain maximal limb length and ensure successful healing. When more of the foot and limb can be preserved, the chances for rehabilitation are improved [16]. Clinical assessment aided by the appropriate diagnostic studies supply the surgeon with valuable information when selecting an amputation site. Anatomic and perioperative issues also need to be addressed when determining the level of an amputation. By careful clinical assessment, use of proper diagnostic modalities, and evaluation of perioperative factors, the surgeon better can select the most favorable amputation site.

References

[1] Krupski WC. Overview of extremity amputations. In: Rutherford RB, editor. Vascular surgery. 5th edition. Philadelphia: WB Saunders; 2000. p. 2175–80.

[2] Armstrong DG, Lavery LA, Harkless LB, et al. Amputation and reamputation of the diabetic foot. J Am Podiatr Med Assoc 1997;87(6):255–9.

[3] Haynes IG, Middleton MD. Amputation for peripheral vascular disease: experience of a district general hospital. Ann R Coll Surg Engl 1981;63(5):342–4.

[4] Campbell WB, Marriott S, Eve R, et al. Factors influencing the early outcome of major lower limb amputation for vascular disease. Ann R Coll Surg Engl 2001;83(5):309–14.

[5] Mandrup-Poulson T, Jensen JS. Mortality after major amputation following gangrene of the lower limb. Acta Orthop Scand 1982;53(6):879–84.

[6] Jamieson MG, Ruckley CV. Amputation for peripheral vascular disease in a general surgical unit. J R Coll Surg Edinb 1983;28(1):46–50.

[7] Gregg RO. Bypass or amputation? Concomitant review of arterial bypass grafting and major amputations. Am J Surg 1985;149(3):397–402.

[8] Rush D, Huston C, Bivins BA, et al. Operative and late mortality rates of above-knee and below-knee amputations. Am J Surg 1981;47(1):36–9.

[9] Tripses D, Pollak EW. Risk factors in healing of below-knee amputation. Appraisal of 64 amputations in patients with vascular disease. Am J Surg 1981;141(6):718–20.

[10] Burgess EM, Matsen FA, Wyss GR, et al. Segmental transcutaneous measurements of PO2 in patients requiring below-the-knee amputation for peripheral vascular insufficiency. J Bone Joint Surg Am 1982;64(3):378–82.

[11] Sethia KK, Berry AR, Morrison JD, et al. Changing pattern of lower limb amputation for vascular disease. Br J Surg 1986;73(9):701–3.

[12] Wutschert R, Bounameaux H. Determination of amputation level in ischemic limbs: reappraisal of the measurement of TcPO2. Diabetes Care 1997;20(8):1315–8.

[13] Bacharach JM, Rooke TW, Osmundson PJ, et al. Predictive value of transcutaneous oxygen pressure and amputation success by use of supine and elevation measurements. J Vasc Surg 1992;15(3):558–63.

[14] Gu YQ. Determination of amputation level in ischaemic lower limbs. ANZ J Surg 2004;74(1–2): 31–3.

[15] Burgess EM, Matsen FA. Determining amputation levels in peripheral vascular disease. J Bone Joint Surg 1981;63(9):1493–7.

[16] Oishi CS, Fronek A, Goldbranson FL. The role of non-invasive vascular studies in determining levels of amputation. J Bone Joint Surg 1988;70(10):1520–30.

[17] Couch NP, David JK, Tilney NL, et al. Natural history of the leg amputee. Am J Surg 1977; 133(4):469–73.

[18] Roon AJ, Moore WS, Goldstone J. Below-knee amputation: a modern approach. Am J Surg 1977;134(1):153–8.

[19] Steinberg FU, Sunroo I, Roettger RF. Prosthetic rehabilitation of geriatric amputee patients: a follow-up study. Arch Phys Med Rehabil 1985;66(11):742–5.

[20] Dowd GS. Predicting stump healing following amputation for peripheral vascular disease using the transcutaneous oxygen monitor. Ann R Coll Surg Engl 1987;69(1):31–5.

[21] McIntyre Jr KE, Berman SS. Patient evaluation and preparation for amputation. In: Rutherford RB, editor. Vascular Surgery. 5th edition. Philadelphia: WB Saunders; 2000. p. 2181–4.

[22] Veith FJ, Gupta SK, Wengerter KR, et al. Changing arteriosclerotic disease patterns and management strategies in lower-limb-threatening ischemia. Ann Surg 1990;212(4):402–14.

[23] Taylor Jr LM, Hamre D, Dalman RL, et al. Limb salvage vs. amputation for critical ischemia: the role of vascular surgery. Arch Surg 1991;126(10):1251–7.

[24] Kald A, Carlsson R, Nilsson E. Major amputation in a defined population: incidence, mortality and results of treatment. Br J Surg 1989;76(3):308–10.

[25] High RM, McDowell DE, Savin RA. A critical review of amputation in vascular patients. J Vasc Surg 1984;1(5):653–5.

[26] Stuck RM, Sage R, Pinzur M, et al. Amputations in the diabetic foot. Clin Podiatr Med Surg 1995;12(1):141–55.

[27] Kalani M, Brismar K, Fagrell B, et al. Transcutaneous oxygen tension and toe blood pressure as predictors for outcome of diabetic foot ulcers. Diabetes Care 1999;22(1):147–51.

[28] Armstrong DG, Lavery LA, van Houtum WH, et al. Seasonal variations in lower extremity amputation. J Foot Ankle Surg 1997;36(2):146–50.

[29] Powell TW, Burnham SJ, Johnson Jr G. Second leg ischemia. Lower extremity bypass versus

amputation in patients with contralateral lower extremity amputation. Am Surg 1984;50(11): 577–80.

[30] Whitehouse FW, Jurgensen C, Block MA. The later life of the diabetic amputee. Another look at the fate of the second leg. Diabetes 1968;17(8):520–1.

[31] Barnes RW, Thornhill B, Nix L, et al. Prediction of amputation wound healing. Roles of Doppler ultrasound and digit photoplethysmography. Arch Surg 1981;116(1):80–3.

[32] Mars M, Mills RP, Robb JV. The potential benefit of pre-operative assessment of amputation wound healing potential in peripheral vascular disease. S Afr Med J 1993;83(1):16–8.

[33] Misuri A, Lucertini G, Nanni A, et al. Predictive value of transcutaneous oximetry for selection of the amputation level. J Cardiovasc Surg 2000;41(1):83–7.

[34] Wagner WH, Keagy BA, Kotb MM, et al. Noninvasive determination of healing of major lower extremity amputation: the continued role of clinical judgment. J Vasc Surg 1988;8(6):703–10.

[35] Adera HM, James K, Castronuovo Jr JJ, et al. Prediction of amputation wound healing with skin perfusion pressure. J Vasc Surg 1995;21(5):823–9.

[36] Durham JR. Lower extremity amputation levels: indications, determining the appropriate level, technique, and prognosis. In: Rutherford RB, editor. Vascular Surgery. 5th edition. Philadelphia: WB Saunders; 2000. p. 2185–213.

[37] Cederberg PA, Pritchard DJ, Joyce JW. Doppler-determined segmental pressures and wound-healing in amputations for vascular disease. J Bone Joint Surg 1983;65(3):363–5.

[38] Keagy BA, Schwartz JA, Kotb M, et al. Lower extremity amputation: the control series. J Vasc Surg 1986;4(6):321–6.

[39] Robbs JV, Ray R. Clinical predictors of below-knee stump healing following amputation for ischaemia. S Afr J Surg 1982;20(4):305–10.

[40] Silverman DG, Rubin SM, Reilly CA, et al. Fluorometric prediction of successful amputation level in the ischemic limb. J Rehabil Res Dev 1985;22(1):23–8.

[41] Dwars BJ, van den Broek TAA, Rauwerda JA, et al. Criteria for reliable selection of the lowest level of amputation in peripheral vascular disease. J Vasc Surg 1992;15(3):536–42.

[42] Lempke RE, King RD, Kaiser GC, et al. Amputation for arteriosclerosis obliterans. Arch Surg 1963;86:406–13.

[43] O'Dwyer KJ, Edwards MH. The association between lowest palpable pulse and wound healing in below knee amputations. Ann R Coll Surg Engl 1985;67(4):232–4.

[44] Wagner WH, Keagy BA, Kotb MM, et al. Noninvasive determination of healing of major lower extremity amputation: the continued role of clinical judgment. J Vasc Surg 1988;8(6):703–10.

[45] Padberg Jr FT, Back TL, Thompson PN, et al. Transcutaneous oxygen (TcPO2) estimates probability of healing in the ischemic extremity. J Surg Res 1996;60(2):365–9.

[46] Criqui MH, Fronek A, Klauber MR, et al. The sensitivity, specificity, and predictive value of traditional clinical evaluation of peripheral arterial disease: results from noninvasive testing in a defined population. Circulation 1995;71(3):516–22.

[47] Hiatt WR, Marshall JA, Baxter J, et al. Diagnostic methods for peripheral arterial disease in the San Luis Valley Diabetes Study. J Clin Epidemiol 1990;43(6):597–606.

[48] Malone JM, Anderson GG, Lakla SG, et al. Prospective comparison of noninvasive techniques for amputation level selection. Am J Surg 1987;154(2):179–84.

[49] Pollak SB, Ernst CB. Use of Doppler pressure measurements in predicting success in amputation of the leg. Am J Surg 1980;139(2):303–6.

[50] Mehta K, Hobson II RW, Jamil Z, et al. Fallibility of Doppler ankle pressure in predicting healing of transmetatarsal amputation. J Surg Res 1980;28(5):466–70.

[51] Welch GH, Leiberman DP, Pollock JG, et al. Failure of Doppler ankle pressure to predict healing of conservative forefoot amputations. Br J Surg 1985;72(1):888–91.

[52] de Graaff JC, Ubbink DT, Legemate DA, et al. Evaluation of toe pressure and transcutaneous oxygen measurements in management of chronic critical leg ischemia: a diagnostic randomized clinical trial. J Vasc Surg 2003;38(3):528–34.

[53] Sarin S, Shami S, Shields DA, et al. Selection of amputation level: a review. Eur J Vasc Surg 1991;5(6):611–20.

[54] Bone GE, Pomajzl MJ. Toe blood pressure by photoplethysmography: an index of healing in forefoot amputations. Surgery 1981;89(5):569–74.

[55] Kram HB, Appel PL, Shoemaker WC. Comparison of transcutaneous oximetry, vascular hemodynamic measurements, angiography, and clinical findings to predict the success of peripheral vascular reconstruction. Am J Surg 1988;155(4):551–8.

[56] Wyss CR, Robertson C, Love SJ, et al. Relationship between transcutaneous oxygen tension, ankle blood pressure, and clinical outcome of vascular surgery in diabetic and nondiabetic patients. Surgery 1987;101(1):56–62.

[57] Ballard JL, Eke CC, Bunt TJ, et al. A prospective evaluation of transcutaneous oxygen measurements in the management of diabetic foot problems. J Vasc Surg 1995;22(4):485–92.

[58] Castronuovo Jr JJ, Adera HMA, Smiedl JM, et al. Skin perfusion pressure measurement is valuable in the diagnosis of critical limb ischemia. J Vasc Surg 1997;26(4):629–37.

[59] Dormandy JA. What is critical leg ischaemia and its pathophysiology? Int Angiol 1993;12: 9–12.

[60] Carter SA, Tate RB. The value of toe pulse waves in determination of risks for limb amputation and death in patients with peripheral arterial disease and skin ulcers or gangrene. J Vasc Surg 2001;33(4):708–14.

[61] Zweifler AJ, Cushing G, Conway J. The relationship between pulse volume and blood flow in the finger. Angiology 1967;18(10):591–8.

[62] Carter SA, Tate RB. Value of toe pulse waves in addition to systolic pressures in the assessment of the severity of peripheral arterial disease and critical limb ischemia. J Vasc Surg 1996;24: 258–65.

[63] Carter SA, Tate RB. The effect of body heating and cooling on the ankle and toe systolic pressures in arterial disease. J Vasc Surg 1992;16(2):148–53.

[64] Bunt TJ, Holloway GA. TcPo2 as an accurate predictor of therapy in limb salvage. Ann Vasc Surg 1996;10(3):224–7.

[65] Zhong J, Seifalian AM, Salerud GE, et al. A mathematical analysis on the biological zero problem in laser Doppler flowmetry. IEEE Trans Biomed Eng 1998;45(3):354–64.

[66] Hauser CJ, Klein SR, Mehringer CM, et al. Superiority of transcutaneous oximetry in noninvasive vascular diagnosis in patients with diabetes. Arch Surg 1984;119(6):690–4.

[67] Hauser CJ, Klein SR, Mehringer CM, et al. Assessment of perfusion in the diabetic foot by regional transcutaneous oximetry. Diabetes 1984;33(6):527–31.

[68] Caligara F, Rooth G, Ewald U. Skin blood flow calculations from transcutaneous gas pressure measurements. Adv Exp Med Biol 1987;220:253–7.

[69] Hauser CJ, Appel PL, Shoemaker WC. Pathophysiologic classification of peripheral vascular disease by position changes in regional transcutaneous oxygen tension. Surgery 1984;95(6): 689–93.

[70] Matsen III FA, Wyss CR, Pedegana LR, et al. Transcutaneous oxygen tension measurement in peripheral vascular disease. Surg Gynecol Obstet 1980;150(4):525–8.

[71] White RA, Nolan L, Harley D, et al. Noninvasive evaluation of peripheral vascular disease using transcutaneous oxygen tension. Am J Surg 1982;144(1):68–75.

[72] Franzeck UK, Talke P, Bernstein EF, et al. Transcutaneous PO2 measurements in health and peripheral arterial occlusive disease. Surgery 1982;91(2):156–63.

[73] Pinzur MS, Stuck R, Sage R, et al. Transcutaneous oxygen tension in the dysvascular foot with infection. Foot Ankle 1993;14(5):254–6.

[74] Quigley FG, Faris IB. Transcutaneous oxygen tension measurements in the assessment of limb ischaemia. Clin Physiol 1991;11(4):315–20.

[75] Wyss CR, Harrington RM, Burgess EM, et al. Transcutaneous oxygen tension as predictor of success after an amputation. J Bone Joint Surg 1988;70(2):203–7.

[76] de Graaff JC, Ubbink DT, Legemate DA, et al. Interobserver and intraobserver reproducibility of peripheral blood and oxygen pressure measurements in the assessment of lower extremity arterial disease. J Vasc Surg 2001;33(5):1033–40.

[77] Padberg Jr FT, Back TL, Hart LC, et al. Comparison of heated-probe laser Doppler and

transcutaneous oxygen measurements for predicting outcome of ischemic wounds. J Cardiovasc Surg 1992;33(6):715–22.

[78] Ratliff DA, Clyne CA, Chant AD, et al. Prediction of amputation healing: the role of transcutaneous pO2 assessment. Br J Surg 1984;71(3):219–22.

[79] Bacharach JM, Rooke TW, Osmundson PJ, et al. Predictive value of transcutaneous oxygen pressure and amputation success by use of supine and elevation measurement. J Vasc Surg 1992;15(3):558–63.

[80] Oishi CS, Fronek A, Golbranson FL. The role of non-invasive vascular studies in determining levels of amputation. J Bone Jt Surg 1988;70(10):1520–30.

[81] Silverman DG, Roberts A, Reilly CA, et al. Fluorometric quantification of low-dose fluorescein delivery to predict amputation site healing. Surgery 1987;101(3):335–41.

[82] Hurford WE, Silverman DG. Evaluation of ischemic extremities by quantative fluorescence assessment. Surg Forum 1982;33:442–3.

[83] Silverman DG, Rubin SM, Reilly CA, et al. Fluorometric prediction of successful amputation level in the ischemic extremity. J Rehabil Res Dev 1985;22(1):23–8.

[84] Klein SG, Hansell JR, Brousseau DA, et al. Fluorescein and microsphere distribution to ischemic skin and bowel. Surg Forum 1985;36:542–4.

[85] Silverman DG, LaRossa DD, Barlow CH, et al. Quantification of tissue fluorescein delivery and prediction of flap viability with the fiberoptic dermofluorometer. Plast Reconstr Surg 1980;66(4):545–53.

[86] Silverman DG, Hurford WE, Cooper HS, et al. Quantification of fluorescein distribution to strangulated rat ileum. J Surg Res 1983;34(2):179–86.

[87] Fairs SL, Ham RO, Conway BA, et al. Limb perfusion in the lower limb amputee: a comparative study using a laser Doppler flowmeter and a transcutaneous oxygen electrode. Pros and Orthotics Intl 1987;11(2):80–4.

[88] Holloway Jr GA, Burgess EM. Preliminary experiences with laser Doppler velocimetry for the determination of amputation levels. Pros and Orthotics Intl 1983;7(2):63–6.

[89] Kvernebo K, Slagsviold CE, Stranden E. Laser Doppler flowmetry in evaluation of skin post-ischaemic reactive hyperaemia. J Cardiovasc Surg 1989;30(1):70–5.

[90] Malvezzi L, Castronuovo Jr JJ, Swayne LC, et al. The correlation between three methods of skin perfusion pressure measurement: radionuclide washout, laser Doppler flow, and photoplethysmography. J Vasc Surg 1992;15(5):823–30.

[91] Adera HM, James K, Castronuovo Jr JJ, et al. Prediction of amputation wound healing with skin perfusion pressure. J Vasc Surg 1995;21(5):823–9.

[92] Holstein P, Sager P, Lassen NA. Wound healing in below-the-knee amputations in relation to skin perfusion pressure. Acta Orthop Scand 1979;50:49–58.

[93] Back TL, Padberg FT, Thompson PN, et al. Probability of successful wound outcome determined by laser Doppler measurements using a heated probe (LDHP). J Vasc Tech 1994;18:67–70.

[94] van den Broek TA, Dwars BJ, Rauwerda JA, et al. Photoplethysmographic selection of amputation level in peripheral vascular disease. J Vasc Surg 1988;8(1):10–3.

[95] Harris JP, McLaughlin AF, Quinn RJ, et al. Skin blood flow measurement with xenon-133 to predict healing of lower extremity amputations. Aust N Z J Surg 1986;56(5):413–5.

[96] Kostuik JP, Wood D, Hornby R, et al. The measurement of skin blood flow in peripheral vascular disease by epicutaneous application of Xenon-133. J Bone Joint Surg 1976;58(6):833–7.

[97] Sejrsen P. Epidermal diffusion barrier to 133Xe in man and studies of clearance of 133Xe by sweat. J Appl Physiol 1968;24(2):211–6.

[98] Moore WS, Henry RE, Malone JM, et al. Prospective use of Xenon Xe 133 clearance for amputation level selection. Arch Surg 1981;116(1):86–8.

[99] Malone JM, Leal JM, Moore WS, et al. The "gold standard" for amputation level selection: xenon-133 clearance. J Surg Res 1981;30(5):449–55.

[100] Durham JR, Anderson GG, Malone JM. Methods of preoperative selection of amputation level. In: Flanigan DP, editor. Perioperative assessment in vascular surgery. New York: Marcel Dekker; 1987. p. 61–82.

[101] Malone JM, Goldstone J. Lower extremity amputation. In: Moore WS, editor. Vascular surgery: a comprehensive review. New York: Grune & Stratton; 1984. p. 909–74.

[102] Holstein P. Level selection in leg amputation for arterial occlusive disease: a comparison of clinical evaluation and skin perfusion pressure. Acta Orthop Scand 1982;53(5):821–31.

[103] Wagner WH, Keagy BA, Kotb MM, et al. Noninvasive determination of healing of major lower extremity amputation: the continued role of clinical judgment. J Vasc Surg 1988;8(6):703–10.

[104] Spence VA, Walker WF, Troup IM, et al. Amputation of the ischemic limb: selection of the optimum site by thermography. Angiology 1981;32(3):155–69.

[105] Raines JK, Darling RC, Buth J, et al. Vascular laboratory criteria for the management of peripheral vascular disease of the lower extremities. Surg 1976;79(1):21–9.

[106] Golbranson FL, Yu EC, Gelberman RH. The use of skin temperature determinations in lower extremity amputation level selection. Foot Ankle 1982;3(3):170–2.

[107] Sizer JS, Wheelock FC. Digital amputations in diabetic patients. Surgery 1972;72(6):980–9.

[108] Porter JM, Baur GM, Taylor Jr LM. Lower extremity amputations for ischemia. Arch Surg 1981;116(1):89–92.

[109] Schwartz JA, Schuler JJ, O'Connor RJ, et al. Predictive value of distal perfusion pressure in the healing of amputation of the digits and the forefoot. Surg Gynecol Obstet 1982;154(6):865–9.

[110] Verta MJ, Gross WS, van Bellan B, et al. Forefoot perfusion pressure and minor amputation for gangrene. Surgery 1976;80(6):729–34.

[111] Baker WH, Barnes RW. Minor forefoot amputation in patients with low ankle pressure. Am J Surg 1977;133(3):331–2.

[112] Nicholas GG, Myers JL, Demuth WE. The role of vascular laboratory criteria in the selection of patients for lower extremity amputation. Ann Surg 1982;195(4):469–73.

[113] Boeckstyns ME, Jensen CM. Amputation of the forefoot. Predictive value of signs and clinical physiological tests. Acta Orthop Scand 1984;55(2):224–6.

[114] Chang BB, Jacobs RL, Darling III RC, et al. Foot amputations. Surg Clin North Am 1995; 75(4):773–82.

[115] Cheng EY. Lower extremity amputation level: selection using noninvasive hemodynamic methods of evaluation. Arch Phys Med Rehabil 1982;63(10):475–9.

[116] Gottschalk FA, Fisher Jr DF. Complications of amputations. In: Rutherford RB, editor. Vascular surgery. 5th edition. Philadelphia: WB Saunders; 2000. p. 2213–27.

[117] Yeager RA, Moneta GL, Edwards JM, et al. Deep vein thrombosis associated with lower extremity amputation. J Vasc Surg 1995;22(5):612–5.

[118] Lind J, Kramhoft M, Bodtker S. The influence of smoking on complications after primary amputation of the lower extremity. Clin Orthop 1991;267:211–7.

[119] Joseph WS. Treatment of lower extremity infections in diabetics. J Am Pod Med Assoc 1992; 82(7):361–70.

[120] McIntyre Jr KE, Bailey SA, Malone JM, et al. Guillotine amputation in the treatment of nonsalvageable lower extremity infections. Arch Surg 1984;119(4):450–3.

ELSEVIER
SAUNDERS

Clin Podiatr Med Surg
22 (2005) 447–467

CLINICS IN
PODIATRIC
MEDICINE AND
SURGERY

Tendon Balancing in Pedal Amputations

Greg D. Clark, DPM, Eric Lui, DPM, Keith D. Cook, DPM*

*Podiatry Service, University Hospital–University of Medicine and Dentistry of New Jersey,
150 Bergen Street, Room A-226, Newark, NJ 07103, USA*

Many circumstances may dictate the need for partial amputation of the foot. Trauma, infection, gangrene, peripheral vascular disease, neuropathic ulcerations, osteomyelitis, and neoplasms are a few of the conditions mandating pedal amputations. Limb salvage is the primary objective and indication for pedal amputation. The goal of any limb-salvage procedure is to provide the patient with a stable, plantigrade foot for ambulation. For foot and ankle surgeons performing a limb-salvage procedure, the first consideration is to determine the level at which the amputation is to be performed.

Higher level amputations, such as below-knee amputations and above-knee amputations, were the procedures of choice until the description of the trans-metatarsal amputation (TMA) by McKittrick et al in 1944 [1]. It has been well documented that more proximal amputations are associated with increased mortality and greater energy expenditure, especially in elderly patients [2–5]. Also, the rate of contralateral limb amputation increases dramatically after a more proximal amputation. When an amputation is performed distally in the foot or ankle, the increased energy expenditure required of a patient when walking is kept to a minimum [6]. Since McKittrick's publication, numerous studies have documented tremendous success in patient outcomes when more distal amputations, such as the TMA, are performed, with healing rates ranging from 44% to 92% [3]. As a result of this success, a TMA is now considered preferable to a below-knee amputation or above-knee amputation because it allows a weight-bearing residuum and has a lower mortality rate [4].

Amputation at the level of Chopart's joint, Lisfranc's joint, or the trans-metatarsal level is met with some skepticism because of potential complications.

Dr. Cook has a financial agreement with Arthrex, Inc, Naples, FL.
* Corresponding author.
E-mail address: cookkd@umdnj.edu (K.D. Cook).

0891-8422/05/$ – see front matter © 2005 Elsevier Inc. All rights reserved.
doi:10.1016/j.cpm.2005.03.003   *podiatric.theclinics.com*

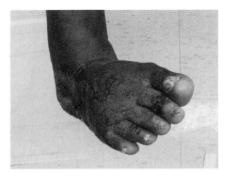

Fig. 1. An adductovarus foot deformity after a fifth metatarsal base resection in which the peroneus brevis tendon was not reattached properly. The residual deformity resulted in recurrent ulcerations to the lateral aspect of the foot.

The greatest complication seen with these distal amputations is the development of equinus or equinovarus deformities [7]. This devastating complication can lead to reulceration or infection and can necessitate further amputations (Fig. 1). Studies indicate that wound failure or higher amputation can occur in 17% to 44% of patients with a TMA [4]. If planned properly, these complications often can be prevented, however, by performing the necessary soft tissue balancing at the time of amputation to keep the foot in a rectus and plantigrade position.

Tendon transfers have long been used as adjunctive procedures to enable stabilization and muscle balancing for patients with neuromuscular diseases. More recently, tendon transfers have played an important role in rebalancing flatfoot and cavus foot reconstruction procedures. With greater understanding of biomechanics, tendon transfers and muscle balancing now are employed as prophylactic measures to prevent the development of future limb deformity. Such is the case when pedal amputations are performed. With the proper use of adjunctive tendon balancing, the foot and ankle surgeon can achieve greater success with limb-salvage techniques. Selection of the appropriate soft tissue balancing comes from an understanding of pedal anatomy and concepts germane to tendon transfers.

Theory and anatomy of pedal tendon transfers

A tendon is composed of approximately 86% collagen (mainly type 1), 1% to 5% proteoglycans, and 2% elastin according to dry weights, with ground substance composing the rest of the tendon. Reticulin provides the bulk of a tendon. A tendon is composed of basic units called *tropocollagen*. The amino acids glycine, proline, and hydroxyproline provide the chemical makeup of tropocollagen. Each tropocollagen molecule is cross-linked with other tropocollagen molecules overlapping by about 10% to 25% of its length forming collagen filaments [7,8]. There are two types of links, intermolecular and intramolecular, which help tendons resist mechanical and enzymatic breakdown. Intramolecular links are formed intracellularly between amino acid chains. They are called *reducible links* and are formed through an enzymatic process. Intermolecular links or mature cross-links are found between tropocollagen molecules. They give a tendon its tensile strength [9].

Collagen filaments combine to form fibrils, which are combined together to form the collagen fiber. A bundle of collagen fibers is invested by endotenon to form a fascicle. The endotenon is a layer of areolar connective tissue that provides for nutrition and innervation. Finally, an aggregate of fascicles forms the structure known as a tendon. The tendon itself is surrounded by epitenon, a one- to two-cell layer of fibroblasts essential for tendon healing. The major vascular supply to a tendon is provided by the paratenon, which is the loose areolar tissue investing the tendon. It also allows for smooth gliding of the tendon with movement.

A four-stage process needs to occur for proper healing after a tendon injury. Stage 1 involves the production of a fibroblastic callus at the site of the tendon injury. This initial inflammatory phase occurs over the first 48 to 72 hours. There is retraction of the tendon ends and an increased vascularity at this site. At this point in tendon healing, after surgical repair, the strength of the sutures outweighs the tensile strength of the healing tendon. Stage 2 involves the production of collagen fibers in a disorganized fashion. The vascularity of the paratenon increases, and there is continued migration and proliferation of fibroblasts into the callus site. Stage 3 involves an increased production of collagen and alignment of the collagen fibers. Passive range-of-motion exercises at this stage stimulate alignment of the collagen fibers, prevent adhesions, and strengthen the site of injury. Stage 4 of healing involves a decrease in vascularity and edema of the tendon. The collagen fibers continue to align and cross-link, increasing the tensile strength of the tendon. Continuing passive range-of-motion exercises stimulate further alignment of the collagen fibers with completion of the alignment process at about 8 weeks. The tendon continues to increase in tensile strength with the formation of cross-linkages.

Blood supply to a tendon is derived from three sources: the myotendinous junction; the osseotendinous junction; and the paratenon, mesotenon, and vincula. Vessels within the collagen fiber bundles travel within the endotenon. At the insertional sites of tendons, the vascular supply of the tendon connects with the osseous vascular supply by communication with the periosteal vessels. Tendons within the foot that have sheaths have a less defined blood supply. The presence of a sheath prevents blood vessels from gaining direct access to the tendon at any given point along its course. Unsheathed tendons have a direct vascular supply by way of the vincula. In most mature tendons, however, most nutrition is derived from synovial fluid diffusion [10,11].

A tendon's position in relation to the axis of a joint determines its effect on the motion about a joint. The closer a tendon is in relation to the joint axis, the more its force acts as a stabilizing force. The farther a tendon is from the joint axis, the more its force acts as a rotary force. In the process of transferring a tendon to compensate for lost function, one must determine the desired effect on motion about a joint.

The following tendons are plantar flexors about the ankle: flexor digitorum longus, flexor hallucis longus, tibialis posterior, triceps surae, peroneus longus, and peroneus brevis. The main plantar flexor is the triceps surae. Extensor digitorum longus (EDL), extensor hallucis longus (EHL), tibialis anterior, and peroneus tertius tendons are dorsiflexors about the ankle with tibialis anterior as the main dorsiflexor. Inversion about the subtalar joint is due mainly to the action of tibialis posterior. Tibialis anterior, triceps surae, flexor hallucis longus, and flexor digitorum longus also assist with inversion of the subtalar joint. Eversion about this joint is due to the peroneus longus, peroneus brevis, EHL, and EDL. Peroneus brevis is the primary evertor of the subtalar joint. Consideration must be given to these basic principles when performing amputations of the foot, specifically proximal amputations, such as TMA and Chopart's amputation.

When performing TMAs, if the fifth metatarsal base is sacrificed, the peroneus brevis tendon should be transferred into the cuboid to prevent a varus deformity of the foot resulting from the unopposed action of tibialis posterior. Likewise, if the insertion of tibialis anterior is compromised, consideration should be given to transferring the tendon into the neck of the talus to prevent equinus deformity resulting from the unopposed action of the triceps surae. If the tibialis anterior tendon is not transferred, tenotomy or lengthening of the Achilles tendon should be strongly considered. Such is the case in a Chopart's amputation in which the insertion of tibialis anterior is sacrificed. A similar situation exists in a TMA in which all insertions of the digital extensors and flexors are lost; this leaves the triceps surae and tibialis anterior as the prime dorsiflexor and plantar flexor of the ankle. The Achilles tendon has a longer moment arm about the ankle joint, and as a result equinus deformities occur as the tibialis anterior is overpowered.

A muscle at 120% of its resting length can produce optimal contraction. At this length, the overlap between the thick and thin filaments within a muscle allows for cross-bridging to occur, generating an optimal contraction. In the resting state, a tendon has a crimped appearance to it. This appearance is due to the ground substance of the tendon. The crimped state of the tendon disappears when a load is applied to the tendon reaching 2% of stretch. At 4% of stretch, the collagen fibers begin to deform. When the load is removed, however, the collagen fibers return to their resting state. At 4% to 8% of stretch, the cross-links between collagen fibers begin to fail, and weaker fibers begin to rupture. The cross-links fail as the collagen fibrils slip past each other. Complete rupture of the tendon occurs at greater than 8% of stretch [9].

When transferring tendons, one must consider transferring same-phase tendons when possible. Same-phase muscle groups are divided into two groups, mainly stance-phase and swing-phase muscles. Stance-phase muscles are tibialis posterior, flexor digitorum longus, flexor hallucis longus, peroneus longus and brevis, and triceps surae. Swing-phase muscles are tibialis anterior, EHL, EDL, and peroneus tertius. Conversion of a swing-phase muscle to a stance-phase muscle or vice versa requires rigorous training of the transferred muscle. Intense physical therapy is employed to attempt muscle conversion; however, success is never guaranteed. With same-phase transfers, adaptation to a new function is possible in 7 to 8 weeks. Out-of-phase transfers that do not convert may be beneficial, however, solely as a result of the resting tension of the muscle.

Muscle power also must be considered in tendon transfers. Muscle strength of grade 4 or more is required for a successful tendon transfer. With the transfer of a tendon, there is a loss of one grade of muscle power. Muscle strength is graded as follows according to the Lovett system [12]:

Grade 5—full resistance at end range of motion
Grade 4—some resistance at end range of motion
Grade 3—motion against gravity only
Grade 2—motion with gravity eliminated
Grade 1—visualized or palpable muscle fasciculations
Grade 0—no muscle contraction noted

Surgical planning

Before any limb-salvage procedure is undertaken, the functional expectations and goals of the patient must be considered. For younger patients with active lifestyles, proximal amputations may be the best option [5]. Recovery periods are shorter, and prosthetic fittings are more tolerable in this patient population. For older or more sedentary patients, amputations that are more distal usually serve best. Addressing individual goals, needs, and expectations of the patient allows the surgeon to plan limb salvage accordingly. The first question to be answered by the surgical team is, "Is the limb salvageable?"

Determination of the ability to salvage a limb incorporates a full workup of the etiology for the amputation, extent of pathology, soft tissue coverage, and neurovascular status. To predict optimal healing, laboratory studies, noninvasive vascular studies, a full nutritional assessment including serum transferrin, total lymphocyte count, total serum protein, and specialty consultations as needed should be obtained before surgical intervention [6]. Certain situations, such as trauma and limb-threatening infections (eg, necrotizing fasciitis), do not afford these luxuries. Often the decision to perform a primary amputation or attempt limb salvage must be made by the surgical team within minutes to hours of initial evaluation. When this pivotal decision has been made, surgical planning is begun. If the limb is deemed nonsalvageable, a proximal amputation, such as a below-knee amputation or an above-knee amputation, is performed. When limb salvage is to be undertaken, a surgical plan must be formulated.

Proper surgical planning is required to determine the level of amputation best suited to the condition at hand because each patient is unique. The optimal level of amputation is a level that allows for maintenance of a functional, propulsive, weight-bearing surface with ability to heal, while preserving as much limb or foot length as possible. It has been documented that increased cardiac workload is related directly to level of amputation with more proximal amputations increasing cardiac demand. Preoperative factors dictating optimal level of amputation include urgency of procedure, consideration of anatomic tendon insertion sites, and whether surgical staging is necessary.

Emergent surgeries for severe trauma and limb-threatening infections do not allow for extensive preoperative workup. In these circumstances, it often is required to stage the procedure into at least two surgical episodes. The primary objective of the initial surgery is to prevent further damage of the extremity by performing an incision and drainage with extensive débridement and bone stabilization when needed. During this initial surgery, it is imperative to maintain as much soft tissue as possible, including plantar and dorsal skin flaps to allow for future wound closure. Intraoperative assessment of vascularity is a valuable indicator of the patient's ability to heal. Also, intraoperative wound cultures are obtained to assist in providing accurate antibiotic coverage. Thought also must be given to the biomechanical implications of the selected level of amputation.

When performing the primary amputation, it is important to keep key tendon insertion sites intact, when possible, to maintain foot function and stability. Loss of insertion sites of the long extensor tendons, tibialis anterior, or peroneal tendons creates gait and structural imbalance leading to debilitating ulcerations and further amputations. If these levels must be sacrificed, tendons should be resected to a healthy level and tagged with nonabsorbable suture for future harvesting and transfer procedures at the time of closure. The surgeon must approach the procedure keeping in mind what tendon balancing will be necessary at the time of wound closure. The functional outcome of a foot after amputation depends not only on adequate removal of irretrievably damaged tissue, but also on muscle rebalancing at the time of amputation or soon afterward [13].

If the initial procedure is performed for frostbite, dry gangrene, or trauma within the 8-hour "golden period," an amputation with primary closure can be performed. This decision usually is made intraoperatively by the appearance of the wound after extensive débridement and irrigation. In this situation, an increased preoperative awareness of maintaining foot function is essential. The surgeon must give extra attention to incision planning in an effort to provide adequate soft tissue coverage for closure and access to key tendon insertion sites for adjunctive tendon balancing procedures. For wounds that are infected, contaminated, or outside of the golden period, the site is packed open and allowed to drain.

The first dressing change is done 36 to 48 hours postoperatively. In this interim, vascular workup is completed, and specialty consultations are obtained, such as vascular and plastic surgery, when indicated. Electromyography and nerve conduction velocities also may be obtained for planning of tendon transfer and rebalancing. If indicated, MRI, CT, or bone scan is obtained to rule out deep space infections or residual osteomyelitis. During the initial dressing change, repeat wound cultures are obtained, and the soft tissue is evaluated for anticipated closure of the wound during the final surgery. After the patient's workup is complete, and medical optimization is reached with wound cultures remaining negative, the patient is brought for revisional amputation with appropriate tendon balancing procedures and wound closure.

Tendon fixation techniques

Tendons that are slated for transfer to a new insertion site must be secured firmly. There are many viable fixation techniques. Ultimately, anatomic location and surgeon preference dictate which method is used.

Tenodesis and anastomosis

Tenodesis is the technique of suturing tendons side by side. An example of this technique is tenodesis of the peroneous longus to the peroneous brevis during a peroneal stop procedure. When performing a tenodesis, care must be taken to roughen the two tendon surfaces being sutured together. Removal of the epitenon on the opposed surfaces improves the success of the procedure. Anastomosis is a similar fixation technique in which the two tendons are fastened together in an end-to-end manner.

Trephine plug

The trephine plug technique involves the creation of a hole within the bone to which the harvested tendon is being transferred. A power or hand trephine can be used for creation of the hole. The tendon is placed within the hole, and the plug of bone is tamped back into place over the transferred tendon. The plug of bone can be secured in place with the use of sutures. The interference screw is a more recent advancement that has eliminated the need for preservation of the trephine bone plug (Fig. 2).

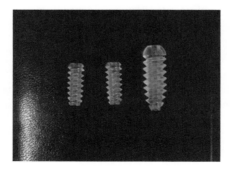

Fig. 2. Bio-Tenodesis Screws (Arthrex, Inc, Naples, Florida). The interference technology allows for secure intratunnel fixation of tendon to bone and eliminates the need for preservation of a bone plug.

Buttonhole

The buttonhole technique involves the passing of a whipped stitched tendon through a drill hole created in the bone. The suture is passed through the skin and threaded through and tied to a button. Padding is placed between the button and the skin to prevent pressure necrosis, and the suture is tied down securing the tendon in place.

Anchors

Tendon anchors are composed of various materials ranging from metals to bioabsorbable components and are available in many different sizes. Some anchors are threaded, and others use a parachute metal prong fixation system. Attached to the anchor is either absorbable or nonabsorbable suture material. The anchor is tamped or screwed into a drill hole created in the bone. The attached suture material is used to secure the tendon, and the suture ends are tied down with the tendon being pulled taut to the bone cortex (Fig. 3). A variation of the tendon anchor is the technique of using a screw and washer. A screw and washer is threaded through the tendon at the point of attachment and tightened down to the bone to serve as fixation.

Tunnels

A tunnel is drilled in the bone, and the tendon is passed through and sutured back onto itself. This technique may be used if there is a sufficient amount of tendon available. The tunnel and sling technique can be used for a variety of tendon transfers, including the Jones tenosuspension procedure.

A variant tendon fixation technique is the three-hole suture method. The three-hole suture technique uses two additional drill holes to allow for passage of suture material. The tendon is passed into the main drill hole and pulled further by

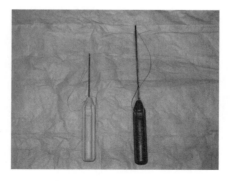

Fig. 3. Variable sizes of soft tissue anchors. The attached suture material is used to suture the tendon onto the bone.

passing the suture back through the two other holes. The sutures are tied down securing the tendon in place.

Tendon with bony insertion involves the transfer of a tendon with a piece of bone harvested from the insertion point. The tendon and attached bone are transferred to a bony deficit that matches the transferred bone. The tendon is secured in place by suturing or using hardware to fixate the transferred bone.

Level of amputation

Digital amputation

Digital amputations are performed routinely as a result of localized trauma, gangrene, or chronic osteomyelitis. Although more readily tolerable in children, adults tend to develop gait abnormalities and instability after digital amputations. Whether a partial or total digital amputation is performed, instability is created secondary to the loss of the long flexor and extensor tendon insertions at the base of the distal phalanx. The long extensor muscles function in swing phase to aid in ground clearance of the forefoot, whereas the long flexors assist in the propulsive phase of gait. Several useful tendon transfers can be considered in digital amputations to afford stabilization of the forefoot during the gait cycle and prevent loss of dorsiflexor strength for ground clearance and progressive equinus deformity.

Partial digital amputations are performed either at the level of the inter-phalangeal joints or through the proximal phalanx. This procedure traditionally is done through a fish-mouth or racquet-type incision. These incisions may be oriented dorsal to plantar or medial to lateral depending on surgeon preference. Dissection is carried through the subcutaneous layers with care to maintain full-thickness skin flaps for closure of the site. Further dissection allows exposure of the long extensor tendon, which is sharply dissected from its insertion to the distal phalanx and tagged with suture to prevent retraction. When the extensor tendon is isolated, bony resection is performed as necessary. Caution is taken to keep the long flexor tendon intact during osseous resection. The long flexor tendon is followed distally to its insertion at the base of the distal phalanx and sharply resected. The distal stump is tagged with suture. When dealing with infected digits, the harvested tendons should be resected to a level of healthy tissue before being tagged with suture material. At this time, completion of the amputation is performed with débridement of all nonviable or infected tissue and bone. The amputation site now is prepared for tendon augmentation, and it is the responsibility of the surgeon to decide if primary closure of the wound is reasonable or if the surgery is to be staged.

In the presence of infection or trauma outside of the golden period, the wound is packed open. At the time of wound closure, the tagged tendons are used to stabilize the digits across the metatarsophalangeal joint, helping to maintain function and balance. There are two ways this stabilization can be achieved:

(1) The flexor and extensor tendons are reattached to the remaining portion of the proximal phalanx, or (2) primary end-to-end anastomosis of the long flexor and extensor tendons is done. Reattaching the tendons to the proximal phalanx may be done with tendon anchors, drill holes, or suture, which involves passing the flexor tendons dorsally over the proximal phalanx, provided that there is enough of the proximal phalanx remaining.

To perform primary anastomosis, a notch first is fashioned at the distal portion of the remaining proximal phalanx using a bone rasp or rotary burr. The tendons are routed in the distal channel where an end-to-end anastomosis is performed with nonabsorbable suture. This technique provides transverse and sagittal plane stability across the metatarsophalangeal joint. Irrigation of the surgical site is performed, and the wound is closed in layers.

Total digital amputation results in the same biomechanical imbalance as partial digital amputation. This imbalance is defined as a metatarsophalangeal joint disarticulation or as a digital amputation with partial metatarsal head resection. The indications for this procedure are identical to the indications of partial digital amputations albeit with a more proximal extent. Amputations at this level require more involved tendon transfer procedures because these transfers provide stabilization across the midtarsal, subtalar, and ankle joint rather than the metatarsophalangeal joint.

The surgical approach to a total digital amputation is identical to that of the partial digital amputation described earlier. A fish-mouth or racquet-type incision is used around the affected digit, allowing enough soft tissue for later closure of the wound. Careful soft tissue dissection is performed to create full-thickness skin flaps and isolate the long extensor tendon of the involved digits. When the long extensor tendon is identified, it is tagged with suture material at its most distal healthy portion and transected. When the tendon is tagged, the digital amputation is completed as a disarticulation of the metatarsophalangeal joint or with a partial metatarsal head resection. After copious irrigation, it is determined if the procedure is to be staged or completed in one setting. When the wound is optimized, tendon balancing is performed.

For each of the harvested extensor tendons, EDL and EHL, there are two transfer techniques that can be used. A common transfer technique for each of these tendons is direct transfer to the corresponding metatarsal neck when a metatarsophalangeal joint disarticulation is performed. Jones [14] and Heyman [15], using EHL and EDL, originally described these techniques for treatment of flexible anterior cavus foot deformity. This transfer is beneficial because of the ease of access and preservation of muscle function. Through the original skin incision, the soft tissue dissection is continued proximally to the corresponding metatarsal neck. The extensor tendon is measured to an appropriate length that allows for proper tensioning and fixation. When the correct length is determined, the tendon is transected at that level and fashioned to the metatarsal neck via a drill hole, anchor, suture, interference screw, or buttonhole as described earlier. Final inspection of tendon tension is evaluated, and the site is irrigated and closed in layers.

In amputations that involve multiple lesser digits or when the metatarsal head is included, a second transfer option is available. Transfer of the EHL to the medial cuneiform maintains the function of dorsiflexion and inversion, whereas transfer of the EDL to the lateral cuneiform provides dorsiflexion and eversion. For multiple digital amputations, it is often beneficial to transfer the entire EDL tendon to the lateral cuneiform as described in the Hibbs procedure because fewer complications are encountered, and function is maintained [16]. This technique is performed through a second skin incision centered over the lateral cuneiform. A 2-cm incision is created with blunt dissection through the subcutaneous layer. Isolation of the EDL tendon is performed just proximal to its separation into individual slips. When the EDL is isolated, it is tagged with suture and transected. Careful dissection is continued deep until the lateral cuneiform is identified. The periosteum is reflected, and the EDL tendon is fixated to the cuneiform under appropriate tensioning; this can be determined by placing the transferred tendon under maximum tension, then releasing the tendon to its relaxed state. The midpoint of this measured distance is the fixation point at which ideal tendon function would occur. The method of tendon fixation is the surgeon's preference. At University Hospital, tendon anchors and interference screws are the preferred methods of tendon fixation (Figs. 4 and 5). Both of the surgical sites are copiously irrigated and closed in surgical layers.

When considering transfer of the EDL to the lateral cuneiform, additional consideration may be necessary for the remaining digits. Instability is created to the remaining intact digits secondary to the loss of the long extensor function. To negate this effect, it may be necessary to perform interphalangeal joint arthrodesis or anastomosis of the long extensor distal stump to the corresponding extensor digitorum brevis tendon.

Transfer of the EHL tendon is performed in a similar fashion by use of a second incision centered over the medial cuneiform. A 2-cm incision is placed parallel to the EHL tendon at the level of the medial cuneiform. Careful soft tissue dissection allows for isolation of the EHL tendon, which is pulled proxi-

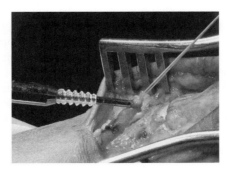

Fig. 4. Use of the Bio-Tenodesis Screw for tendon fixation. The tendon and screw are inserted into the predrilled hole in the bone. Tensioning of the tendon can be adjusted by moving the screw and suture, which passes through the screw and has been looped around the tendon, proximally or distally.

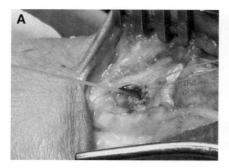 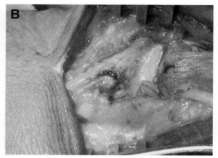

Fig. 5. Use of the Bio-Tenodesis Screw for tendon fixation. (*A*) After insertion of the tendon and screw, the suture ends are hand tied together. (*B*) The tied suture ends are cut. The tendon and screw are well secured into the bone.

mally, introducing the severed distal stump into the proximal incision site. Dissection is continued deep to the level of bone with care to avoid the dorsalis pedis artery. The periosteum is reflected, and the EHL tendon is appropriately tensioned and fixated to the medial cuneiform. An alternative option is to isolate the tibialis anterior tendon and perform a side-to-side anastomosis of the EHL to the tibialis anterior along with fixation of the EHL tendon to the medial cuneiform. After confirming proper tensioning of the transferred tendon, the surgical sites are irrigated and closed in layers.

All of the aforementioned procedures are beneficial in providing a stable foot and maintaining muscle function when digital amputations are necessary. The extent of soft tissue and bony injury often necessitates a more proximal level of amputation.

Transmetatarsal amputation

The TMA originally was described as an operation to salvage the foot for ambulation and as an alternative to higher level amputations, which have an increased mortality rate. The three indications for performing a TMA were (1) gangrene of the digits, (2) stabilized distal infection of the foot, and (3) neuropathic foot with infected ulcers [1]. This procedure also is useful in the presence of failed digital amputations or extensive forefoot trauma. Since the first description of the TMA, tremendous success has been documented for this procedure with healing rates reaching 92% [3]. Despite the high success rate with TMAs, development of equinus or equinovarus deformity postoperatively can be a devastating complication.

TMAs sacrifice the insertion sites of EHL, EDL, and sometimes peroneus tertius. An imbalance of muscle pull is created across the ankle joint as the gastrocnemius-soleus complex greatly overpowers the only remaining ankle joint dorsiflexor, tibialis anterior. This muscle imbalance creates the equinus deformity commonly seen after a TMA. The equinus deformity is compounded by a subtalar joint imbalance that also is created with TMA. The inversion pull of the tibialis anterior and tibialis posterior overpower the opposing eversion pull of the peroneous brevis and longus, creating a varus position of the rearfoot. In addition to these deformities, Chrzan et al [17] further described the loss of the "rigid beam effect" secondary to the release of the intrinsic foot muscles and plantar fascia, causing an early heel-off and increased pressures on the TMA stump.

During gait, TMA ankles use approximately 70% of available static range of motion of dorsiflexion, whereas intact ankles use 90% of available dorsiflexion [2]. This "functional equinus" is a key contributor to skin breakdown and re-ulceration of the TMA stump. With proper use of tendon balancing at the time of the amputation, these complications can be prevented.

The surgical approach to a TMA is through a fish-mouth incision placed proximal to the affected region of the forefoot. Care is taken to maintain a large, full-thickness plantar flap for closure of the site. Osteotomies are made through each of the metatarsals at a level that removes all infection and allows for wound closure. The osteotomies are fashioned in a manner to maintain the metatarsal parabola and create a plantar bevel to reduce risk of pressure ulcerations. Medial and lateral beveling also is performed to the first and fifth metatarsals. It is important to maintain as much metatarsal length as possible to reduce the mechanical advantage of the Achilles tendon. When the amputation site is optimal, closure is performed in layers, and appropriate tendon balancing procedures are performed.

Several surgical treatment options are available to restore balance across the subtalar and ankle joints in conjunction with TMA procedures. These tendon-balancing procedures are aimed at bringing the ankle and subtalar joints into a neutral position to prevent future stump breakdown and additional surgery. The tibialis anterior tendon and the Achilles tendon are the main focus for restoring balance across the rearfoot joints. A split tibialis anterior tendon transfer (STATT) allows rebalancing by reducing the inversion strength of the tibialis anterior, while strengthening the eversion pull across the subtalar joint. Complete transfer of the anterior tibial tendon laterally restores the dorsiflexor pull from the anterior compartment to counteract the opposing pull of the Achilles and posterior tibial tendons. Whether performing a STATT or a complete tibialis anterior transfer, a three-incision approach is necessary. The first incision is placed at the insertion site of the tibialis anterior. Blunt dissection allows isolation of the tibialis anterior tendon that is followed to its insertion. A second incision is placed on the anterior lower leg just proximal to the superior extensor retinaculum. Soft tissue dissection is carried to the level of the tendons, and the tibialis anterior tendon is identified. At this time, either the lateral half of the tibialis anterior tendon or the entire tendon is harvested from its osseous insertion and pulled into the second incision site. Finally, a third incision is placed on the dorsal aspect of the foot centered over the cuboid or lateral cuneiform, where dissection is carried down to the periosteum. The harvested tibialis anterior tendon is routed beneath the extensor retinaculum and introduced into the third incision site. At this time, the tendon is tensioned as described previously and fixated to the cuboid when performing a STATT or the lateral cuneiform when performing a total tendon transfer. The tendon is fixated to the bone via the surgeon's preferred fixation technique. All three surgical sites are irrigated and closed in layers.

Achilles tendon lengthening or Achilles tenotomy is performed to weaken the pull of the posterior muscles. Lengthening the Achilles tendon reduces driving force, stride length, and shear force, all of which contribute to ulcer development [18]. After lengthening of the Achilles tendon, the gastrocnemius-soleus complex loses the ability to decelerate the forward momentum of the leg during midstance and the ability for heel lift, both acting to shorten stride length. When the stride length shortens, less pressure and force is transmitted to the distal aspect of the foot. Studies by Armstrong et al [19] and Mueller et al [20] showed that peak pressure decreased by approximately 27% after an Achilles tendon lengthening.

The surgical approach is based on surgeon preference. For tendon lengthening, either an open "Z" or tongue-in-groove lengthening is performed via a posterior incision over the Achilles tendon, or a percutaneous triple hemisection can be used as described by Hoke [21]. When performing a TMA, the authors prefer to perform an Achilles tenotomy via a single lateral or medial incision. After completion of the amputation, a single 1-cm linear incision is made adjacent and parallel to the Achilles tendon approximately 3 cm proximal to the insertion site. Blunt dissection is used to create a soft tissue plane anterior and posterior to the Achilles tendon with care to avoid the sural nerve and medial neurovascular bundle. A no. 15 scalpel blade is introduced into the incision site anterior to the Achilles tendon and turned 90°. Gentle pressure is applied against the tendon, and the foot is dorsiflexed. Immediate release of the Achilles tendon should be felt with an audible "crunch" and a noticeable increase in ankle dorsiflexion. The surgical site is inspected for any remaining intact tendon fibers that are released if found. Copious irrigation is performed, and the skin is closed with nylon suture (Fig. 6).

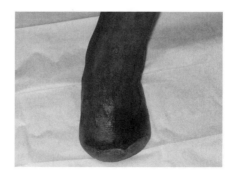

Fig. 6. A 44-year-old man 1 year status post transmetatarsal amputation with Achilles tenotomy. A flexible plantigrade foot was achieved.

Lisfranc's amputation

Lisfranc's amputation is similar in surgical technique to the TMA in terms of incision planning. The dorsal incision is made just distal to Lisfranc's joint, and, if possible, a long plantar flap is maintained. Lisfranc's joint is identified and disarticulated. Consideration must be made for tendon transfers resulting from the loss of the insertions of the peroneus brevis and peroneus longus tendons. When the fifth metatarsal base is disarticulated, the peroneus brevis tendon should be transferred to the cuboid. Split transfer or transfer of the entire tibialis anterior tendon laterally also may be performed. An Achilles tendon lengthening or tenotomy also should be performed with this proximal amputation. These two tendinous procedures decrease the likelihood of the development of an equinovarus deformity. Some surgeons perform a tibialis posterior tenotomy in conjunction with a Lisfranc's amputation to prevent frontal plane deformity. Further long-term results are needed, however, to determine the effectiveness of this procedure.

When performing any amputation involving the forefoot or midfoot, as much length as possible should be preserved. There is a greater chance of developing an equinus deformity with more proximal amputations as the Achilles tendon gains a mechanical advantage. Achilles tenotomy or lengthening is always performed. Consideration should be given to the arches of the foot—medial, lateral, and transverse. The medial longitudinal arch is composed of the calcaneus, talus, navicular, cuneiforms, and first three metatarsals. The lateral longitudinal arch is composed of the cuboid, calcaneus, and fourth and fifth metatarsals. Care should be taken to preserve the integrity of the transverse arch of the foot located at the level of the cuneiforms and cuboid. With Lisfranc's amputation, the transverse arch is disrupted, resulting in a varus deformity. Chopart's amputation is proximal to the transverse arch and avoids a varus deformity by creating a level weight-bearing surface [22].

Chopart's amputation

Chopart was the first to describe the midtarsal joint amputation (or Chopart's amputation) [23]. A common complication during its inception was equinus deformity leading to ulceration of the stump and further amputation. MacDonald [24] and Bingham [25] later modified the procedure, by transferring the tibialis anterior tendon into the neck of the talus to combat equinus deformity. With time, lengthening of the Achilles tendon also was advocated to prevent the equinus deformity. Lengthening of the Achilles tendon has been shown in studies to decrease plantar pressures, preventing ulcerations in neuropathic feet (Fig. 7) [19]. This is an important fact in a Chopart's amputation because of the loss of the extensor tendons.

Other modifications to Chopart's amputation include transfer of the extensor tendons into the neck of the talus and resecting the prominences of the distal talus and calcaneus. The advantage of Chopart's amputation over Lisfranc's am-

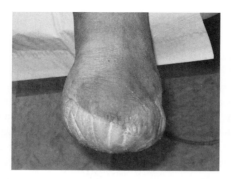

Fig. 7. A patient status post Chopart's amputation with Achilles tenotomy. The amputation site is healed, and the rectus foot is accommodated with custom-made shoes. A lateral plantar ulcer developed secondary to hypertrophic bone production.

putation is the elimination of the resulting equinovarus deformity. The tendon insertions of the tibialis posterior and anterior are eliminated, preventing frontal plane deformity. More distal amputations are beneficial, however, for the reasons stated earlier.

A fish-mouth incision is made with the apices of the fish mouth located at the level of the midtarsal joint. The incisions are extended distal to the midtarsal joint and across the dorsal and plantar aspects of the foot with preservation of a longer plantar flap. The incisions are deepened to bone, and the tibialis anterior tendon is dissected free. Soft tissue dorsal to the midtarsal joint is elevated allowing for identification and access to Chopart's joint. When the joint is identified, the foot is sharply disarticulated at this level. All tendons except for the tibialis anterior tendon are pulled distally and transected as proximally as possible. The tendons are allowed to retract.

The tibialis anterior tendon is transferred into the neck of the talus. Next the Achilles tendon is lengthened or a snap tenotomy is performed. The authors' preferred method is the snap tenotomy, which ensures that equinus deformity does not recur, as is possible with an Achilles tendon lengthening. The plantar flap is remodeled if necessary and brought up to the dorsal skin. The wound is closed in layers.

Syme amputation

The original Syme amputation was described for salvage of the gangrenous and nonsalvageable diabetic limb. This procedure involves amputation through the ankle joint with preservation of the heel fat pad. This technique provides a stable and viable stump that can be fitted easily with a prosthesis and avoids stump irritation commonly seen with transtibial amputations. Some studies have shown that the Syme amputation is less metabolically demanding than proximal (transtibial) and distal (TMA, Lisfranc) amputations [26,27]. This is an important fact considering that most amputations occur in diabetics with an already compromised cardiovascular system. Disarticulation at the ankle joint provides a longer lever arm for propulsion, resulting in a less metabolically demanding gait pattern compared with that seen in midfoot amputations [5]. Midfoot amputations still are preferred, however, over the more proximal below-knee amputation.

The surgical approach involves making an incision over Chopart's joint from the medial to the lateral aspect of the foot. The incision is carried toward the plantar aspect of the foot with preservation of the heel flap. When the ankle joint is disarticulated, the medial and lateral malleoli are resected and planed to provide a flat surface. The fat pad of the heel is brought dorsally to provide cushion for the amputation site. Originally the procedure was a two-stage procedure: The first stage involved the primary amputation, and the second stage involved remodeling of the malleoli and closure of the wound. This procedure was performed in stages to avoid wound infection and failure of the amputation. Pinzur [28] since has shown, however, that the Syme amputation can be performed as a single-stage procedure.

Complications

There are inherent complications to any surgical procedure, including infection, swelling, pain, scar formation, and loss of function. Specific complications are associated with tendon transfers. Improper tensioning of the transferred tendon may lead to overcorrection or undercorrection of the deformity, rendering the transfer unsuccessful or useless. Piazza et al [29,30] have shown that a large error in tensioning is required to have transfer failure.

Complications also may arise from tendon fixation. As mentioned earlier, many different techniques may be used to fixate a tendon to bone or another tendon. Each of these techniques has advantages and disadvantages. Fixation failure results in a failed tendon transfer. It has been shown that suture anchors typically fail at the suture material and not at the anchor itself [31]. The appropriate fixation technique for the specific tendon transfer along with the strongest suture material always should be used to obtain optimal fixation and results. Although amputations and the tendon transfers performed along with them are associated with complications, the authors believe that failure to attempt the proper tendon transfer can have even greater consequences. The proper tendon transfer with optimal fixation needs to be performed to decrease the chance of complications and to achieve a successful outcome.

Postoperative course

Patients undergoing any procedure involving a tendon transfer should be immobilized in a posterior splint postoperatively. This immobilization prevents

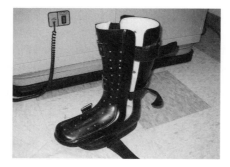

Fig. 8. After lower extremity amputation, the limb should be accommodated with custom-made braces or shoes to support the extremity in function. A custom-made Charcot Restraint Orthotic (Langer Inc., Deer Park, New York) walker is pictured.

possible disruption of the tendon from its new insertion site. The authors recommend immobilization and non–weight bearing for 2 to 4 weeks to allow for proper tendon healing. Gentle passive range-of-motion exercises may be initiated as tolerated during postoperative week 3 to propagate tendon healing and mobilization. At postoperative week 4, the cast or splint may be discontinued, and the patient may be advanced to partial weight bearing in a pressure-relief boot with the assistance of crutches or a walker. At this stage in recovery, physical therapy is initiated to strengthen the transferred tendon and increase the patient's lower extremity range of motion after immobilization. If an out-of-phase tendon transfer has been performed, physical therapy is used to re-educate the transferred muscle. Finally, appropriate orthoses and prostheses may be employed as necessary to prevent further ulceration or to support the lower extremity in function (Fig. 8).

Summary

Pedal amputations are an essential part of the armamentarium of most foot and ankle surgeons. An amputation should not be viewed as a destructive procedure, but as a limb-salvaging and, in some cases, a lifesaving procedure. The goal of pedal amputation is to provide the patient with a stable, plantigrade foot for ambulation. When performing a pedal amputation, consideration always must be given to the use of tendon balancing to provide the stable, plantigrade platform on which ambulation occurs. Failure to balance the foot properly may result in increased deformity and more proximal amputations.

The foot and ankle surgeon must understand lower extremity biomechanics and the mechanical function of each tendon involving the foot. Specific tendon transfers, lengthenings, or tenotomies are required at each level of pedal amputation. At a minimum, residual equinus deformity after a TMA or more proximal

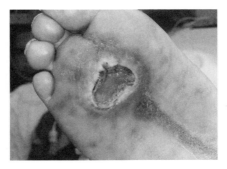

Fig. 9. A 36-year-old diabetic man with a history of right foot partial second ray resection. Postoperatively, the patient developed a plantar forefoot ulcer, which was treated unsuccessfully for 10 months with local wound care and offloading. After conservative treatment failed, an Achilles tendon lengthening was performed, and GraftJacket (Wright Medical Technology, Inc, Arlington, Texas) was applied to the ulcer.

pedal amputation needs to be prevented with an Achilles tendon lengthening or tenotomy. Achilles tendon lengthening also has proved beneficial in healing distal forefoot ulcerations (Figs. 9–11).

When performing a tendon transfer, care must be taken to tension the transferred tendon properly to provide maximal function. A variety of reattachment techniques are available to the surgeon. The technique used should be based on anatomic location and surgeon comfort and preference. After a successfully healed pedal amputation, the foot should be able to be accommodated with custom-made bracing or shoes. Physical therapy also may be required to help the patient adjust to his or her new gait pattern.

Although a pedal amputation may be psychologically devastating to a patient, it is usually a necessary limb-salvaging procedure. Proper tendon balancing needs to be performed by the foot and ankle surgeon to help prevent

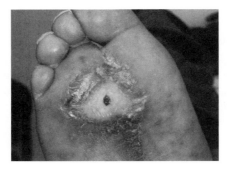

Fig. 10. The same patient as in Fig. 9 at 6 weeks postoperatively. The ulcer is almost entirely healed.

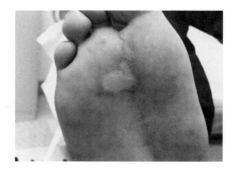

Fig. 11. The same patient as in Fig. 9 at 6 months ostoperatively. The ulcer has healed completely without reoccurrence.

more proximal amputations, allow the patient to ambulate, and maintain a functional lifestyle.

References

[1] McKittrick L, McKittrick J, Risley T. Transmetatarsal amputation for infection or gangrene in patients with diabetes mellitus. Ann Surg 1949;130:826–30.
[2] Garbalosa J, Cavanagh P, Wu G, et al. Foot function in the diabetic patients after partial amputation. Foot Ankle Int 1996;17:43–8.
[3] Hosch J, Quiroga C, Bosma J, Peters E, Armstrong D, Lavery L. Outcomes of transmetatarsal amputations in patients with diabetes mellitus. J Foot Ankle Surg 1997;36:430–4.
[4] Mueller M, Allen B, Sinacore D. Incidence of skin breakdown and higher amputation after transmetatarsal amputation: implications for rehabilitation. Arch Phys Med Rehabil 1995;76: 50–4.
[5] Pinzur M, Wolf B, Havey R. Walking pattern of midfoot and ankle disarticulation amputees. Foot Ankle Int 1997;18:635–8.
[6] Pinzur M, Kaminsky M, Sage R, et al. Amputations at the middle level of the foot. J Bone Joint Surg Am 1986;68:1061–4.
[7] Kannus P. Structure of the tendon connective tissue. Scand J Med Sci Sports 2000;10:312–20.
[8] Lin T, Cardenas L, Soslowsky L. Biomechanics of tendon injury and repair. J Biomech 2004; 37:865–77.
[9] Curwin S. Biomechanics of tendon and the effects of immobilization. Foot Ankle Clin 1997;2: 371–89.
[10] Fenwick S, Hazleman B, Riley G. The vasculature and its role in the damaged and healing tendon. Arthritis Res 2002;4:252–60.
[11] Benjamin M, Ralphs J. Tendons and ligaments—an overview. Histol Histopathol 1997;12: 1135–44.
[12] Wright W. Muscle training in the treatment of infantile paralysis. Boston Medical and Surgical Journal 1912;167:567.
[13] Hansen S. Salvage or amputation after complex foot and ankle trauma. Orthop Clin North Am 2001;32:181–6.
[14] Jones R. The soldier's foot and the treatment of common deformities of the foot. BMJ 1916; 1:749.
[15] Heyman C. The operative treatment of clawfoot. J Bone Joint Surg 1932;14:335.
[16] Hibbs R. An operation for clawfoot. JAMA 1919;73:1583.

[17] Chrzan J, Giurini J, Hurchik J. A biomechanical model for the transmetatarsal amputation. J Am Podiatr Med Assoc 1993;83:82–6.

[18] Barry DC, Sabacinski KA, Habershaw GM, Giurini JM, Chrzan JS. Tendo Achilles procedures for chronic ulcerations in diabetic patients with transmetatarsal amputations. J Am Podiatr Med Assoc 1993;83:96–100.

[19] Armstrong D, Stacpoole-Shea S, Nguyen H, Harkless L. Lengthening of the Achilles tendon in diabetic patients who are at high risk for ulceration of the foot. J Bone Joint Surg Am 1999;81: 535–8.

[20] Mueller M, Sinacore D, Hastings M, Strube M, Johnson J. Effect of Achilles tendon lengthening on neuropathic plantar ulcers. J Bone Joint Surg Am 2003;85:1436–45.

[21] Hoke M. An operation for the correction of extremely relaxed flat feet. J Bone Joint Surg 1931; 13:773–83.

[22] Armstrong D, Hadi S, Reyzelman A. Limb salvage with Chopart's amputation and tendon balancing. J Am Podiatr Med Assoc 1999;89:100–3.

[23] Christie J, Clowes CB, Lamb DW. Amputations through the middle part of the foot. J Bone Joint Surg Br 1980;62:473–4.

[24] Macdonald A. Chopart's amputation. J Bone Joint Surg Br 1955;37:468.

[25] Bingham J. The surgery of partial foot amputation. In: Arnold E, editor. Prosthetic and orthotic practice. London: Edward Arnold; 1970. p. 141.

[26] Waters R, Perry J, Antonelli D, Hislop H. Energy cost of walking of amputees: the influence of level of amputation. J Bone Joint Surg Am 1976;58:42–6.

[27] Pinzur M, Gold J, Schwartz D, Gross N. Energy demands for walking in dysvascular amputees as related to the level of amputation. Orthopedics 1992;15:1033–7.

[28] Pinzur M. Syme ankle disarticulation in peripheral vascular disease and diabetic foot infection: the one stage versus two-stage procedure. Foot Ankle Int 1995;16:124–7.

[29] Piazza S, Adamson R, Moran M, Sanders J, Sharkey N. Effects of tensioning errors in split transfers of tibialis anterior and posterior tendons. J Bone Joint Surg Am 2003;85:858–65.

[30] Piazza S, Adamson R, Sanders J, Sharkey N. Changes in muscle moment arms following split tendon transfer of tibialis anterior and tibialis posterior. J Bone Joint Surg Am 2003;85:858–65.

[31] Barber F, Herbert M, Richards D. Sutures and suture anchors: update 2003. Arthroscopy 2004; 20:985–90.

ELSEVIER
SAUNDERS

Clin Podiatr Med Surg
22 (2005) 469–484

CLINICS IN
PODIATRIC
MEDICINE AND
SURGERY

Complications of Pedal Amputations

James P. Sullivan, DPM, FACFAS, DABPS*

*Podiatric Medicine and Surgery, Department of Orthopaedics,
Jersey Shore University Medical Center, Neptune, NJ, USA*

Pedal amputation in and of itself is often a salvage procedure. As such, amputation often results in an eventful postoperative course, fraught with a variety of challenging complications. These complications often result in the need for revision surgery. The goal of an amputation procedure is to achieve a definitive level at which the amputation will heal, and the foot will remain healed with no further breakdown for the life of the patient. Reasons for a complicated healing course after pedal amputation include vascular, infection, orthopedic, neurologic, metabolic, psychosocial, and medicolegal components. Cases of patients who undergo multiple procedures to heal an amputation often include many and sometimes all of these factors.

Preoperative planning and perioperative decision making are tantamount to successful amputations of the foot. This article discusses the reasons leading to complications status post partial amputation of the foot. Understanding these causes often minimizes a challenging course of healing, which all podiatric surgeons encounter after pedal amputations. Box 1 groups some of these complications into various categories.

Infection

Partial foot amputations often are performed as a staged procedure, initially in the presence of severe infection. Ascending infections, such a necrotizing fasciitis or plantar space infections, often result in a multistaged procedure. After initial open amputation and evacuation of infection, wounds usually are left open

---

* 2130 Route 35, Suite 312, Building C, Sea Girt, NJ 08750.
E-mail address: jpsdpm@verizon.net

0891-8422/05/$ – see front matter © 2005 Elsevier Inc. All rights reserved.
doi:10.1016/j.cpm.2005.03.004
podiatric.theclinics.com

Box 1. Factors related to post–pedal amputation complications

Infection
- Osteomyelitis
- Necrotizing fasciitis
- Premature wound closure

Vascular
- Arterial insufficiency
- Edema

Orthopedic
- Transfer lesions
- Biomechanical breakdown
- Muscle-tendon imbalance

Dermatologic
- Hyperkeratosis
- Stasis dermatitis
- Verrucous hyperplasia

Neurologic
- Insensate foot
- Charcot neuroarthropathy
- Stump neuroma
- Phantom pain

Metabolic
- Poor nutritional status
- Diabetic foot disease
- Renal insufficiency

Psychosocial
- Noncompliance
- Obesity
- Depression
- Smoking
- Low income
- Poor living situation (nursing home or inadequate home care)

Medicolegal
- Cannot obtain informed consent for appropriate procedure
- Risk for medical malpractice lawsuits

to drain. The wound may then be closed and revised at a later date after the infection is under control. Although some surgeons await three negative wound cultures before closure, ideally a negative quantitative tissue culture is the true indication that the wound is ready for closure, from an infection standpoint. This test is not always readily available at all institutions, and using this criterion for closure is not always clinically practical. Closure often is performed when the wound infection appears to be clinically resolved, with no purulence, no fever, normal white blood cell count, and evidence of presence of abundant granulation tissue. These parameters vary among individual clinicians and patients.

Aggressive sensitivity-based antibiosis is crucial to successful amputation. Adequate débridement of infected and nonviable tissue allows for successful closure after amputation. Aggressive preoperative antibiotic treatment even without signs of infection is often warranted [1].

After initial amputation, open wounds often are treated with vacuum-assisted closure and pulsed lavage to combat bacterial wound colonization [2]. Vacuum-assisted closure often promotes the formation of abundant granulation tissue. Presence of granulation tissue suggests the wound's capacity to heal by secondary intention, delayed primary closure, or skin grafting if necessary.

Postoperative infection after amputation is often due to premature wound closure or inadequate, underaggressive surgical débridement and evacuation of the infection. When treating osteomyelitis, it is often difficult to distinguish infected bone from pathology such as Charcot arthropathy, osteoporosis, and renal osteodystrophy. Soft or nonbleeding bone does not always indicate osteomyelitis. Diagnostic imaging is often helpful in determining the extent of bone that needs resection. Underaggressive bone resection leads to dehiscence and infection of the incision several weeks after closure.

The severity of necrotizing skin infections often is underestimated at the time of initial débridement and primary open amputation. The skin and wound edges may necrose rapidly, even in a patient with adequate arterial flow to the foot. Boggy, violaceous skin, which has a foul odor after the amputation, is suspicious for full-thickness necrotizing infection. This infection must be treated aggressively with wide expansile excision when it is recognized and diagnosed. Failure to contain the infection, with local aggressive débridement and antibiotics, may result in the need for a more proximal amputation, such as open distal ankle disarticulation or below-knee amputation.

The use of antibiotic-impregnated resorbable beads has been helpful in treating infection before and at closure. These beads are helpful with the management of dead space, after resection of bone, such as a metatarsal head resection. Drainage through the incision is common for several weeks after closure over the beads. This drainage usually subsides when the beads have resorbed completely radiographically and should not be misdiagnosed as infection or seroma.

After lower extremity bypass graft, edema and hyperemia may place physiologic and mechanical stress on a closed amputation incision. Light compression over the incision may decrease the chance of dehiscence and wound complication. Nonpurulent infection of poorly perfused soft tissue and bone often changes after vascular reconstruction, resulting in a productive purulent drainage. For this reason, definitive amputation and wound closure is best performed no sooner than 3 days after reperfusion of the limb.

Minimizing postamputation infection greatly reduces postoperative morbidity and decreases the need for revision procedures and staged surgical closure. After open amputation, it is sometimes necessary to allow wounds to heal by secondary intention, often expedited by vacuum-assisted wound closure. Plastic surgical consultation and skin grafting is sometimes the best approach, rather than to trying to close an amputation that does not have the capacity to heal by primary closure.

Necrotizing fasciitis and severe skin and soft tissue infections often appear much worse after the initial débridement. Serial débridement with aggressive resection of soft tissue often results in the need to revise the osseous resection level to provide a clean soft tissue envelope with which to close over the bone. It often takes several days of observation and local wound care until the definitive level of amputation may be determined.

Vascular complications

One of the most common reasons for pedal amputation is arterial insufficiency. Appropriate preoperative determination of suspected viability is helpful in determining the level at which the amputation should occur. Complication related to vascular necrosis indicates that the site for amputation may have been poorly selected, or the tissue handling during the procedure may have been too aggressive and traumatic, resulting in local tissue necrosis [3]. Suturing a poorly perfused wound closed with too much tension across the suture line results in local tissue necrosis and possible failure of amputation at that level. Gentle reapproximation of the skin edges facilitates small vessel arterial flow to the wound edges. Loosely tied sutures and even Steri-strips alone are sufficient to assist with successful healing, without risking ischemia to the wound edges. Placement of taught horizontal mattress bolster sutures often leads to local ischemic tissue necrosis at the wound edges.

Noninvasive vascular studies and transcutaneous oxygen tension greater than 30 mm Hg merely *suggest* the level at which an amputation is *likely* to heal. Pulse volume recordings, segmental pressure readings, and duplex ultrasound all are recommended, and vascular surgical consultation is often necessary to access the severity and anatomic location of the ischemia [4]. Generally an ankle-brachial index of 0.45 or less is a poor prognostic indicator that a partial foot amputation does not have the capacity to heal. This reading is often falsely elevated in the presence of sclerotic calcified vessels. Digital toe pressures are valuable predictors of postamputation viability of toe and ray amputations. No study can show an absolute end point beyond which failure or healing is ensured [5].

The best indicator to decide which level is most likely to heal is the clinical appearance of the particular wound before and during surgery. The presence of at least one palpable pedal pulse usually warrants attempted definitive partial foot amputation closure, before more aggressive vascular surgical intervention.

Often, after amputation for dry gangrene, well proximal to the necrotic line of demarcation, the amputation does not have adequate tissue perfusion to support

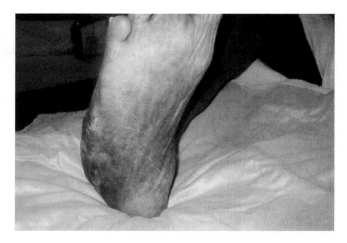

Fig. 1. Verrucous hyperplasia is noted after delayed closure of resected fifth ray.

healing, and the incision line becomes necrotic. Even after successful vascular reconstruction, the tissue still may not heal, and revisional surgery may be inevitable, necessitating a more proximal amputation than originally anticipated. A screening system based on distal runoff vessel patency as shown on preoperative angiography has been successful in determining the level at which the amputation should occur with the greatest chance of healing [6].

Venous insufficiency and lymphedema may complicate healing, leading to difficulty with wound closure. The physical presence of interstitial edema may cause a tamponade effect on the small vessels, causing arterial compromise and ischemia to the distal soft tissues. Postamputation compressive therapy is often underused, resulting in edema and eventual dehiscence and incision complications. Verrucous hyperplasia may form on the stump site because of inadequate edema control (Fig. 1). Stasis dermatitis may develop secondary to venous insufficiency after in situ bypass grafting, which sacrifices the great saphenous vein, contributing to postoperative edema and potential dehiscence.

Patients with calcified vessels often present a hemostasis challenge, which must be managed with postoperative compression for at least 48 hours to avoid collection of hematoma. Patients with pharmacologic and pathologic coagulopathy present with a similar scenario, and the use of closed suction drains, hemostatic agents, and wound packing can decrease the chance of complication after pedal amputation.

Orthopedic complications

Perhaps the most technique-based complication related to pedal amputation includes poor biomechanical weight-bearing surface, resulting in greater mechanical stress and ultimate tissue breakdown. Well-fitted prosthetic and orthotic devices in an extra-depth shoe may accommodate a poor biomechanical result and avoid failure at the amputation site. Sharp uneven bone spurs and exostoses often result in stump failure. Sporadic regrowth of long bones after adequate and smooth resection is seen in Charcot patients and in pediatric patients with an open growth plate. After transfemoral amputation on patients who have not reached skeletal maturity, polytetrafluoroethylene felt caps have been suggested to prevent continued bone growth at this level [7]. Epiphysiodesis may be considered in the metatarsals in these patients after partial foot amputation.

Muscle tendon imbalance occurs, at least to some degree, with most partial foot amputations. Segmental resection of medial, lateral, or distal pedal components results in functional instability, with one muscle group overpowering another. Medial resection results in overpowering by the lateral and anterior muscle groups. This overpowering eventually results in a valgus position and ulceration medially in an insensate foot. Lateral resection results in a biomechanical advantage to the plantar and medial structures. This situation may progress to the development of an acquired clubfoot or equinovarus deformity (Fig. 2). The insensate plantar lateral foot is vulnerable and subject to chronic ulceration. Resection of the distal pedal segment results in equinus if Achilles tenotomy or tendon transfer is not performed. Muscle and tendon imbalance results in a flexible, reducible instability, which ultimately becomes a fixed deformity. If it is not addressed appropriately and treated quickly by tendon-balancing surgery, arthrodesis and major reconstructive surgery become nec-

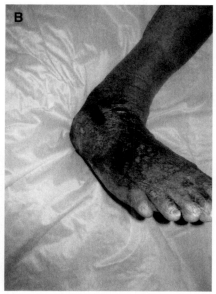
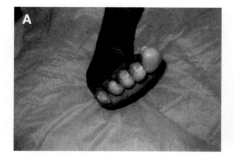

Fig. 2. (*A* and *B*) Adductovarus rotation is noted 1 year after resection of the base of the fifth metatarsal and loss of function of the peroneus brevis.

essary to avoid failure of amputation at this level. Specific illustrations of this phenomenon are discussed subsequently, relative to the level at which the amputation is performed.

Tendon transfers are often necessary to correct muscle-tendon imbalance. Adductovarus rotation after resection of the fifth ray and functional loss of the peroneus brevis may progress to an acquired clubfoot deformity (see Fig. 2). If this deformity is recognized and diagnosed in a timely fashion, it can be corrected with posterior medial release and transfer of the posterior tibial tendon, through the interosseous membrane, into the cuneiforms. When tendon-balancing procedures are successful, more aggressive bone reconstruction may be averted. Bracing of these deformities is a viable option in an inactive patient who is not likely to ambulate frequently, but rarely allows the patient to return to normal functional capacity.

Hallux amputations

Loss of plantar flexor function causes an apropulsive gait and is to be expected after great toe amputation. This amputation may shift undue stress to the lesser metatarsals, resulting in stress fractures, transfer lesions, and ulcerations. Because the extensor hallucis longus tendon insertion is lost with hallucal amputation, diminished forefoot dorsiflexion strength may cause or exacerbate an existing ankle equinus deformity. Transfer of the long extensor to the head or neck of the first metatarsal may avoid this complication. Rigid second hammer toe may develop, causing dorsal or distal lesions, which may ulcerate and lead to infection (Fig. 3).

Limited digital amputation

An isolated digital amputation may result in transverse plane deformity and deviation of the adjacent digit (Fig. 4). Resection of the second toe often results in hallux valgus as the hallux abducts in the transverse plane toward the third toe (Fig. 5). Toe spacers, incorporated into an orthosis or a removable digital prosthesis, may prevent this complication. When multiple toes are amputated, any remaining digits and their relative metatarsals may be subject to an increased plantar pressure and subsequent ulceration. Extensor tenotomy or arthroplasty of the affected digit reduces the likelihood of this complication.

Pan-digital amputation

Amputation of all the digits 1 through 5 at the metatarsophalangeal joint preserves the natural metatarsal parabola, essentially equalizing the submetatarsal forefoot pressures. The loss of long extensor functional strength may result in an equinus deformity. Rather than individually transferring extensor tendons to all five metatarsal necks, a more practical transfer of the extensor hallucis longus tendon to the first metatarsal helps to balance the power of the triceps surae.

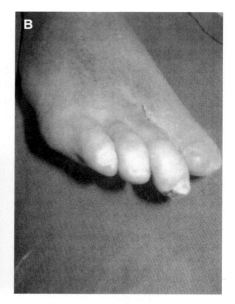

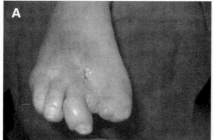

Fig. 3. (*A* and *B*) After resection of the first toe and second partial ray, the third toe is rotated in adductovarus causing pressure ulceration at the distal lateral tip of the distal phalanx. The toe is rotated in the frontal, transverse, and sagittal plane. This ulcer became infected, and the toe required amputation.

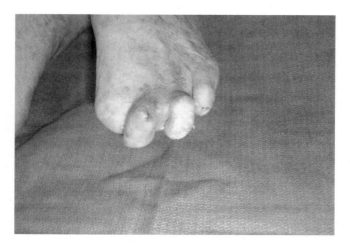

Fig. 4. The first and fourth toes have been amputated. As a result of intrinsic muscle imbalance, there is rigid contracture of the toes with distal and dorsal pressure lesions.

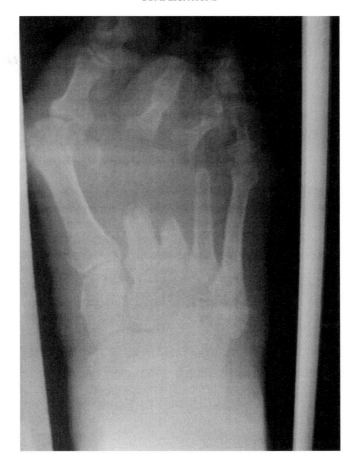

Fig. 5. The metatarsal parabola is poorly constructed, and this patient developed a large submetatarsal ulcer. Imbalance after the resection of the second and third metatarsal heads has facilitated dislocation of the first metatarsophalangeal joint.

Limited ray resections

When a ray resection heals, and the patient begins to ambulate, the most common complication is transfer lesions [8]. First and fifth ray resections often produce a biomechanically sound plantigrade weight-bearing surface. This resultant foot also is fitted easily with an orthotic with a pressure moldable custom foam filler for the amputated ray. Central ray resection is more likely to result in adjacent transfer lesions and tissue breakdown. Adjacent metatarsal stress fractures are a complication of ray resections. These fractures are often asymptomatic in patients with neuropathy and Charcot (Fig. 6).

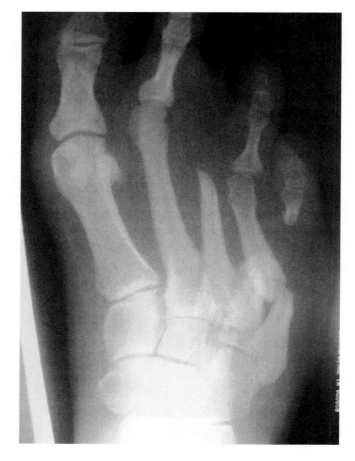

Fig. 6. Asymptomatic stress fracture of the fourth metatarsal after partial resection of the adjacent third and fifth metatarsals.

Distal transmetatarsal amputation

The most common biomechanical reason for complication at this level is a poor metatarsal parabola. The first metatarsal should be beveled from proximal-plantar-medial to distal-dorsal-lateral. The second metatarsal should be beveled from plantar-proximal to dorsal-distal and neutral in the transverse plane. It should be the longest metatarsal in the parabola. The third, fourth, and fifth metatarsals should be beveled from dorsal-distal-medial to plantar-proximal-lateral in a stepwise fashion. The fifth metatarsal should be shorter than the fourth, which should be shorter than the third. A significant deviation from this formula may result in failure of the stump, either plantar or distally. Revision of the metatarsal parabola is often necessary, and preoperative planning is paramount. Intraoperative fluoroscopy is helpful in establishing a sound parabola when gross visualization of all of the metatarsals is not likely. After bone resection, all jagged and sharp edges must be removed by a rongeur or bone rasp. Any area of uneven pressure often complicates the amputation when the patient begins to bear weight. Stump failure and tissue breakdown can be avoided if careful and diligent steps are taken to follow these guidelines.

Early signs of complication should be treated with appropriate wound care and offloading the area in question. If the complication worsens, the parabola should be formally revised in the operating room as described earlier. Converting a distal amputation to a more proximal amputation at the metatarsal bases is often the best approach to definitive, long-lasting healing.

Proximal transmetatarsal amputation

Whether amputation is revisional or primary at the base of the metatarsals, the same principles hold true relating to the metatarsal parabola. Because of the loss of function of the long extensors and the tibialis anterior tendon, an Achilles tendon lengthening or tenotomy should accompany any proximal transmetatarsal amputation. If this is not performed, the foot eventually progresses to an equinus deformity, and distal stump breakdown and failure is inevitable. Transfer of the tibialis anterior tendon into the medial cuneiform is recommended in addition to the lengthening. If healthy tendon tissue is sparse after débridement, the tendon may be transferred more proximally, to the navicular or the talar neck. At the authors' institution, an Achilles procedure always is performed whenever the resection level is proximal to the midshaft of the metatarsals.

Distal and plantar stump failure, in the presence of a well-fashioned parabola, usually is attributed to contracture and equinus deformity, resulting in weight bearing on the stump, rather than the plantar foot. This complication is treated initially with a percutaneous Achilles tenotomy. The tenotomy can be performed in the outpatient, office, or clinic situation under local anesthesia. Thorough understanding of any distal bypass procedures avoids any interruption of the restored blood flow, and the percutaneous method should be discussed with the vascular surgeon preoperatively. If this release is not sufficient to yield a plantigrade foot, delayed tendon transfer as described earlier may be necessary. In some cases, the soft tissue release and tendon transfer are unsuccessful, and ankle or pantalar arthrodesis may be the only method by which a plantigrade foot is achieved.

Chopart (midfoot) amputation

Transosseous midtarsal and Chopart disarticulation are controversial, but when successful, they often are preferred to a below-knee amputation. A propulsive gait may be facilitated with the proper prosthesis and well-made shoe. Amputation at this level is poorly tolerated and prone to ulceration in the neuropathic population. There is an intense pressure load on this stump, which often results in tissue breakdown without proper bracing to offload the plantar foot. Failure usually is noted plantar rather than distal because of the shortened lever arm with these types of amputation.

Symes amputation

Symes described a foot amputation at the ankle level by disarticulation and resection of the medial and lateral malleoli. Special care must be taken to preserve the subcalcaneal fat pad. This procedure is a better alternative to below-knee or transtibial amputation for a select group of patients. Posttraumatic patients with sensate fat pads and no signs of infection are best suited for Symes amputation. A significant limb-length discrepancy is to be expected; however, it is much less significant than with a below-knee amputation. Pinzur et al [9] reported 31 of 38 well-healed amputations that did not require additional revision surgery and tolerated a foot prosthesis well 9 years after amputation. In the insensate fat pad, there is the risk of neuropathic ulceration resulting from the weight-bearing stress concentrated on the relatively small surface area of the retained fat pad. Premature weight bearing postoperatively contributes to dehiscence and stump failure, and patient compliance is vital to the viability of the stump. Although this procedure is not commonly performed, it is a viable alternative to more proximal amputation in the right patient population.

Pirigoff amputation

Pirigoff described foot amputation rather than below-knee amputation after World War I for posttraumatic patients. This procedure involves the excision of the talus and partial resection of the calcaneus, with primary tibiocalcaneal arthrodesis. The same complications as for the Symes amputation can be expected. Additionally, the possibility of malunion or nonunion of the arthrodesis must be considered [5].

Neurologic complications

Local neurologic complications include sensory deficit after nerve transection, amputation stump neuromas, and phantom limb syndrome. Neuropathic ulceration may occur in the insensate foot. After amputation, a smaller surface area is responsible for bearing the same body weight, which the entire foot supported before amputation. This is a recipe for plantar tissue breakdown, ulceration, and infection. Orthotic management is paramount in the insensate foot after amputation.

Patients with Charcot neuroarthropathy are at great risk of complication after amputation. The combination of sensory neuropathy, loss of proprioception, increased load, and muscle imbalance result in breakdown of plantar skin and intra-articular pathologic fractures and dislocation. Evidence of midfoot Charcot deformity may be noted subsequent to partial ray resection as a result of imbalance and worsening sensory neuropathy.

Many sensory nerves are transected during amputation, and the skin levels distal to the transaction are often insensate. This situation results in greater risk for tissue breakdown, ulceration, and infection leading to stump failure. Special care and meticulous tissue handling may preserve the sensory innervation to the distal stump, decreasing the potential for tissue breakdown resulting from neuropathy.

Amputation stump neuromas are among the most common complications of amputation. They occur similar to neuromas after a neurectomy or traumatic nerve transection. Patients may experience pain, hypersensitivity, and paresthesias at the distal amputation level. Diagnosis is often by palpation and the presence of a Tinel sign with tingling on compression and palpation of the neuroma [10]. While performing an amputation, it is important to handle nerve tissue gently. Care should be taken to handle only the nerve distal to the amputation site. Similar to the manner in which tendons are resected, the nerve should be pulled taut and transected proximally with a sharp scalpel; this facilitates the retraction of the nerve ending proximal to the amputation site and away from the weight-bearing surface of the foot. Interdigital and intermetatarsal nerves usually retract and are buried gently in the intrinsic musculature of the foot. The transected nerve may become adherent to a scarred and fibrotic wound bed, causing an increase in size and symptoms associated with the neuroma [11]. Scissors should not be used to transect the nerve because they may cause crushing of the nerve. Crush injury to the nerve by surgical or blunt trauma results in fibrosis and scar tissue formation, which may result in amputation stump neuroma in the foot. Excessive postoperative pressure and friction on the amputation site may result in the formation of a neuroma [12].

After any amputation, the phantom limb syndrome may occur. The painful radiation and paresthesias may be perceived in a phantom limb distribution [11]. This phenomenon may include a burning or crushing sensation in the distribution of the amputated limb. The patient also may "forget" that the limb has been amputated and try to put pressure on the nonexistent extremity, causing loss of balance and trauma related to falling [13].

Metabolic and nutritional complications

After amputation in diabetic patients, healing is complicated if the patient's serum glucose is not well controlled. Hyperglycemia results in neuropathy, vascular insufficiency, immunopathy, and renal insufficiency [14]. Nephropathy results in the spilling of protein into the urine, creating albumin deficiency. Closure of wounds and performing the definitive amputation procedure is best delayed until the metabolic and nutritional status of the patient is maximized to provide the best healing environment for the stump site. Ideally the serum albumin should be at least 3 g/dL [5].

Psychosocial complications

Many patients experience severe depression after amputation, even of a single digit. Elderly patients are especially prone to depression because feelings of mortality and an incomplete body result in bitterness, sadness, and anger. Preoperative counseling and a supportive physician-patient relationship may decrease the extent of the depression. Thorough discussion and explanation of the rationale for and expected outcome of the procedure is important. A good preoperative comfort level and understanding of the proposed procedure often helps to avoid the onset of depression after amputation. Signs of depression should be evaluated, and psychiatric consultation should be considered when necessary. Postamputation grievance support groups are available in many hospitals and communities and may be valuable to this type of patient. A strong family support system often helps patients adjust after amputation and can be proactive in the patient's participation in physical therapy and rehabilitation. If one senses preoperatively that the patient may be at risk for depression after amputation, psychiatric counseling should be encouraged before amputation. Special care should be taken to ensure that a definitive level of amputation is planned because many patients cannot tolerate the emotional stress of multiple procedures, which may be perceived as the "widdling away" of their body. Depression may result in decreased caloric intake, poor nutritional status, substance abuse, and inactivity. All of these factors contribute to the complication rate after foot amputation.

Smoking and tobacco use result in a higher incidence of postoperative complications. Smoking cessation 4 to 8 weeks before surgery significantly reduces the complication rate after surgery [15]. Patients must be counseled and made aware of the deleterious effect that tobacco use has on the healing of their amputation.

Noncompliance in this patient population is voluntary and involuntary. Although some patients do not care for their incisions and wounds because of apathy, ignorance, and denial, others simply cannot care for their amputations for many reasons. Patients with a low income may not be able to afford home nursing care or inpatient rehabilitation facilities that are often necessary to care for a partially amputated foot during the postoperative convalescence period. Transportation may not be accessible for follow-up even in a free clinic or outpatient setting. Poor living situations without family or friends to care for these patients often contribute to the failure of amputations.

Medicolegal complications

Amputation should not be viewed as failure of appropriate medical care delivery. In the current society, however, there must be someone to blame for the loss of limb. The surgeon trying to salvage the limb is often the person that the patient and family members hold responsible for their loss. It is often difficult to obtain informed consent for amputation in this situation. The surgeon often is given limited consent in which minimal resection of tissue is agreed upon. This is a difficult situation because the surgeon may be forced to be too conservative with the débridement and selected level of amputation. Select ray amputations may be consented, when the patient would best be served with a transmetatarsal amputation. Compromising surgical decision making is never a good idea, but it is sometimes unavoidable. It is important to explain to the patient and family members the reason why the more proximal procedure must be done. Documentation of all personal and telephone conversations relating to these challenges is necessary and appropriate. Although the surgeon may not be able to convince the patient to allow an Achilles tenotomy in conjunction with a proximal transmetatarsal amputation, he or shse may be the person the patient holds responsible when the stump breaks down owing to "iatrogenic" equinus deformity 6 months after amputation. All patients undergoing partial foot amputation should be informed that they might need further revisional surgery after this particular amputation.

Summary

Partial foot amputations and revision and closure of such are some of the most challenging cases handled by all foot and ankle surgeons. Preoperative planning, timing of surgery, and intraoperative decision making are key aspects to successful and uncomplicated healing of foot amputations. Every patient has variable and individual complication risks unique to each case. The goal of complete healing, with no need for revision of the amputation for the life of the patient, often may seem lofty, but this is how each individual case should be approached. A healthy fear and understanding of the possible complications for each procedure help the foot and ankle surgeon to achieve this goal more often than not.

References

[1] Edmonds M, Foster A. The use of antibiotics in the diabetic foot. Am J Surg 2004;187:255–85.
[2] Mustoe T. Understanding wounds: a unifying hypothesis on their pathogenesis and implications for therapy. Am J Surg 2004;187:655–705.
[3] Abramson D. Vascular disorders of the extremities. 2nd edition. New York: Harper & Row; 1962. p. 46–51.
[4] Teodoresci VJ, Chen C, Morrissey N, Faries PL, Marin ML, Hollier LH. Detailed protocol of ischemia and the use of non-invasive vascular laboratory testing in diabetic foot ulcers. Am J Surg 2004;187:755–805.
[5] Sage R. Limb salvage. In: Banks AS, Downey MS, Martin DE, Miller SJ, editors. 3rd edition. McGlamry's comprehensive textbook of foot and ankle surgery. 3rd edition. Philadelphia: Lippincott Williams & Wilkins; 2001. p. 1617–32.
[6] Gu YQ. Determination of amputation level in ischemic lower limb. Aust N Z J Surg 2004;74: 31–3.
[7] Tenholder M, Davids JR, Gruber HE, Blackhurst DW. Surgical management of juvenile amputation overgrowth with a synthetic cap. J Pediatr Orthop 2004;24:218–26.

[8] Gianfortune P, Pulla RJ, Sage R. Ray resections of the insensitive or dysvascular foot: a critical review. Journal of Foot Surgery 1985;24:103–7.

[9] Pinzur MS, Morrison C, Sage R. Syme's two stage amputations in insulin requiring diabetics with gangrene of the forefoot. Foot Ankle 1991;11:394–6.

[10] Herndon JH. Neuromas. In: Green DH, Hethchkiss RN, editors. Operative hand surgery. 3rd edition. New York: Churchill Livingstone; 1993. p. 1387–400.

[11] Botte MJ. Traumatic neuromas of the foot and ankle. Foot Ankle Clin 1998;3:71–113.

[12] Herndon JH, Hess AV. Neuromas. In: Gelberman RG, editor. Operative nerve repair and reconstruction. Philadelphia: JB Lippincott; 1991. p. 1525–40.

[13] Berke G. Lower extremity prosthetics. In: Myerson M, editor. Foot and ankle disorders, vol 1. Philadelphia: WB Saunders; 2000. p. 505–6.

[14] Burch W. Endocrinology for the house officer. 2nd edition. Baltimore: Williams & Wilkins; 1988.

[15] Lindstrom D, Wladis A, Linder S, Nasell H, Adami J. Preoperative cessation of smoking seems to reduce frequency of complications. Lakartidningerv 2004;101:1920–2.

ELSEVIER
SAUNDERS

Clin Podiatr Med Surg
22 (2005) 485–502

CLINICS IN
PODIATRIC
MEDICINE AND
SURGERY

Prosthetic Management of the Partial Foot Amputee

Peter P. Yonclas, MD*, Casey J. O'Donnell, DO

*Department of Physical Medicine and Rehabilitation, New Jersey Medical School–UMDNJ,
Suite 3100 DOC, 90 Bergen Street, Newark, NJ 07109, USA*

Partial foot amputations provide advantages and challenges to the patient confronting loss of limb and the rehabilitation team. The partial foot amputation offers the potential for retention of plantar load-bearing tissues, which are uniquely capable of tolerating the forces involved in weight bearing; this can allow the patient to ambulate with or without a prosthesis. Because of the complexity of the foot-ankle complex, the multiple types of partial foot amputations encountered, and the high incidence of vascular and neuropathic compromise in patients with amputations, the rehabilitation team must be keenly aware of several issues. First, the rehabilitation team must be attentive to the individual needs of the patient and his or her adjustment to the loss. In addition, the rehabilitation team must take into account the patient's changes in gait and the subsequent alteration in weight-bearing surfaces, the functional level of the partial foot amputee, and the alignment of the prosthesis. This article identifies the unique challenges found in this patient population and reviews the indications and options available for prosthetic foot management.

Goals of prosthetic management of the partial foot amputee

The rehabilitation of a patient with limb loss requires the skills of many health care professionals to ensure that all needs are being met. Ideally, all of the health care specialists—the surgeon, the physiatrist, the prosthetist, the physical therapist, and the social worker—who are involved in the care of the patient should

---

* Corresponding author.
E-mail address: yonclape@umdnj.edu (P.P. Yonclas).

function together as a team. With their combined experience and knowledge, they can provide the best care possible for the patient who must undergo prosthetic rehabilitation.

The goals of prosthetic management of any patient with limb loss are to maintain function, prevent further deformity, and restore as much independence as possible. When encountering a new amputee, it also is important to remember that the goal of the prosthesis is not simply to replace a lost body part. The objective is also to address the patient's specialized needs and, perhaps more importantly, their expectations. To ensure that the most comfortable, cosmetic, and functional prosthesis has been designed is only part of the goal for prosthetic rehabilitation. The health care providers also should be cognizant of how the patient is adapting to the loss of their limb and how to help facilitate their acceptance of their altered function [1].

Physiatric prosthetic evaluation

Given the complexities of partial foot amputations and prosthetic choices, the surgeon ideally should refer a postamputation patient to a qualified physiatrist almost immediately after the surgery. Although the patient would not be fitted for the prosthesis on the initial visit, an early physiatric evaluation serves to mobilize the rehabilitation team and provides a continuum of care for the patient. The physiatrist can play an integral role in helping with pain management, wound healing, edema control, dwelling modification, and evaluation for durable medical equipment. During the course of wound healing, the physiatrist also can be used to promote general strengthening and cardiovascular conditioning, which prepare the patient for the increased workload associated with ambulating with a prosthesis.

When the incision has healed fully, and the residual limb is satisfactory for weight bearing, the surgeon should inform the physiatrist so that arrangements can be made to create a permanent prosthesis. The physiatrist works closely with the prosthetist to ensure not only the proper construction and fit of the prosthesis, but also to ensure that the needs and expectations of the patient are addressed. The physiatrist also monitors for skin changes suggesting abnormal pressure distribution. This monitoring is crucial because if a patient were to wear an improperly fitting prosthesis, poorly distributed pressure could lead to skin breakdown, infection, and further amputation.

After delivery of the prosthesis, the physiatrist continues to monitor the patient indefinitely. At first, a physiatrist may wish to see the patient on a weekly basis to ensure proper fitting of the prosthesis, evaluate gait dynamics, and assess the patient's stability with and without assistive devices. When the physiatrist and prosthetist feel comfortable that the patient and the prosthesis are working in harmony, follow-up visits usually are spaced 1 month or more apart. Eventually a physiatrist may feel comfortable evaluating the patient only semiannually or annually. These long-term follow-up appointments are crucial not only to monitor for the aforementioned situations, but also to assess for normal wear and tear of the prosthesis. A patient's life is a dynamic situation, and continuous assessment is necessary to ensure that the patient always has the appropriate prosthetic and adaptive equipment for his or her lifestyle.

Definitions of partial foot amputations

Partial foot amputations include a variety of different anatomic levels that result in different functional capabilities for the amputee. Types of amputations include toe or digit amputations, ray resections, and metatarsal amputations and surgical disarticulation at Chopart's and LisFranc's levels (Fig. 1). Toe amputations commonly involve disarticulations at the interphalangeal or metatarsophalangeal joints. Ray resections involve removal of the toe and the associated metatarsal. LisFranc's amputation is at the tarsometatarsal joints and involves separating the cuboid and cuneiform bones from the metatarsal bones of the forefoot. Chopart's amputation involves a disarticulation at the midtarsal joints, where the talus and navicular bones and the calcaneus and cuboid bones are separated.

In addition to amputations at the level of the forefoot, amputations at the ankle joint include the Boyd and Syme's amputations. These procedures often are performed because they may provide a distal weight-bearing surface for the amputee rather than proceeding to a more proximal transtibial amputation. Most experts believe that rehabilitation of a patient after an ankle disarticulation is far simpler than rehabilitation of a patient after a transtibial amputation [2]. The Boyd amputation involves a talectomy with a shift of the calcaneus for

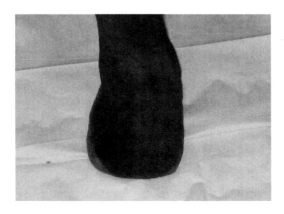

Fig. 1. LisFranc surgical disarticulation.

talocalcaneal arthrodesis, which leaves more of the calcaneus intact. As opposed to the Boyd amputation, Syme's amputation does not lengthen the distal residual limb as much. In the Syme procedure, the amputation involves removal of the distal projections of the tibia and fibula at the talocrural joint and the forefoot. In this procedure, the fat pad of the heel is preserved, then attached to the distal tibia. The Boyd and Syme's amputations must have an intact and healthy heel before proceeding.

Overview of the effects of a partial foot amputation on gait

To understand better the impact of partial foot amputations on the amputee, one first must understand the purpose and components of normal gait. Saunders et al [3] defined the functional task of walking as the translation of the center of gravity through space in the manner that requires the least energy expenditure. The gait cycle is considered to be the period of time between any two identical events in the walking cycle. Each cycle of gait can be divided into the stance and swing phase. The stance phase is considered to be the time when the foot is in contact with the ground and constitutes approximately 60% of the gait cycle. The swing phase denotes the time when the foot or residual leg is in the air and constitutes the remaining 40% of the gait cycle. The stance phase consists of approximately five subphases that involve the acceptance and transfer of weight—initial contact, loading response, midstance, terminal stance, and preswing. The swing phase consists of three phases that involve the propulsion of the advancing leg—initial swing, midswing, and terminal swing subphases.

During the normal gait cycle, the foot-ankle complex serves three main functions: (1) to decrease the impact forces, (2) to maintain equilibrium, and (3) to transmit the propulsive forces of the lower extremity muscles. In early stance phase, the foot-ankle complex must decrease the shock that is transmitted to the knee and hip and absorb the energy from initial contact; this is accomplished partly by the plantar fat pad and through pronation of the subtalar joint and flattening of the arches with eccentric contraction of the tibialis anterior, posterior tibialis, flexor hallucis, and flexor digitorum longus muscles [4,5]. The length of the foot also serves as a lever arm that helps rock the center of gravity of the body over the knee to preserve the elevation of the body at terminal stance. In late stance phase, the foot and lower leg transmit the propulsive forces generated by the gastrocnemius-soleus complex to drive the body forward.

When the foot-ankle complex is unable to compensate for deficits in motion or structure because of amputation, gait abnormalities may develop that can compromise potentially vulnerable tissue. Pinzur et al [6] described the functional relationship between gait velocity and the level of amputation of the foot. As the amputation level becomes more proximal, the gait shows a characteristic reduction in velocity and the step length of the sound leg with a simultaneous increase in energy demand and vertical load on the sound limb.

Typically the weight progression of the stance leg is from heel to toe, with the foot serving as a lever arm for energy absorption and propulsion. In a patient with a partial foot amputation, this progression is altered or absent, and the patient is unable to propel the body with the foot during toe-off [7]. As the foot becomes shorter, the ground contact and the functional lever arm of the foot decrease. The residual limb must compensate for this loss of length by working harder and absorbing more of the ground reaction force, which creates more stress [8]. In addition, there is an abrupt weight transfer to the opposite limb, which can reduce step length and velocity, resulting in an increase in the energy demands of ambulation. This can lead to increased loads being absorbed on the sound limb with possible increase in degenerative joint changes and subsequent risk of future skin breakdown [9].

Prosthetic prescription

Although a prosthetic prescription for a partial foot amputation may not be as difficult as for more proximal amputations, there are still some essential areas that must be covered. First, the physiatrist, or prescribing physician, should be aware of the patient's expectations to ensure that the prosthesis is used to its full advantage. Second, the physician should know if he or she is evaluating the patient for a temporary or permanent prosthesis. In most cases of a partial foot amputation, the prescription is for a permanent prosthesis. The third decision to make is in choosing the type of material for the prosthesis or insert. Carbon fiber is lightweight, durable, and energy efficient, but also is the most expensive. Thermal molded plastic is cheap and easily adjusted, but is heavier than carbon fiber. Shoe inserts can be made of a variety of foam materials, each with their own pros and cons. In general, when referring to a physiatrist, it is best to describe the patient's daily lifestyle activities, weight-bearing status, and surgical complications or abnormalities in the prescription. This information enables the physiatrist and prosthetist to create the most suitable prosthesis for the patient.

Overview of prosthetic components

There are a wide variety of options for the different levels of partial and full foot amputations currently available to the rehabilitation team. Because of the variability in amputation level, sensitivity of the residual limb, patient activity level, and patient expectations, no single prescription can be used for each level of amputation. Instead a prosthetic prescription should follow the goals of bearing weight only on the nontender, viable portion of the foot (typically the hind foot) and minimizing weight bearing especially on the late phase of stance on the distal stump [7]. Generally, as the amputation level becomes more proximal, and the higher the level of activity, the more complex and costly is the prosthetic. A basic overview follows of common options available for some of the most common pedal amputation levels.

Toe amputations

Amputation of the hallux and lesser digits is reserved for cases involving localized gangrene and osteomyelitis in the phalanges. A single toe amputation generally does not alter normal gait or stance phase, but it may cause increased deformity in the remaining toes. Typically, amputation of a single digit still allows the amputee to maintain a normal walking speed. The amputee notices a difference, however, with higher level activities, such as running or jumping. A patient with a great toe amputation may develop a limp as the speed of ambulation increases because the first toe is no longer able to provide additional propulsion during the toe-off phase of gait. In this situation, an appropriate toe filler can be used to prevent collapse of the toe box. The filler prevents the toe box from irritating the skin of the residual foot and improves the shoe's appearance [10]. Toe fillers consist of a soft foam material, such as a foam or a vulcanized lastomer, which fills up the void left in the shoe. Alone, the fillers provide little functional advantage except for the prevention of toe migration. With the loss of the second toe, there is an increased risk of a severe hallux valgus deformity as the great toe is abducted toward the third digit. This deformity can be limited by the insertion of an appropriate toe filler that can be matched to the color of the patient's skin.

The effects of loss of a digit can be more significant in terms of weight distribution in patients with vascular or neuropathic compromise in the amputated and the contralateral foot [11]. Typically with lesser digit amputations, there is little effect on how the weight is distributed. After hallux amputations, the peak pressure on the sole of the foot becomes greater under the first metatarsal head and lesser under the remaining metatarsal heads and toes [12]. Lavery et al [12] compared great toe amputations with the intact contralateral feet. They found that not only was there increased wear on the ipsilateral metatarsal heads, but also there was evidence of new breakdown on the contralateral foot. These patients may need extra-depth or custom-molded shoes and molded accommodative inserts [13].

Molded accommodative inserts may help to decrease the stress on the dysvascular foot in two ways. First, the inserts are made of soft materials that compress on contact with the ground. This compression helps to decelerate the foot at initial contact and decreases the shear on the foot in early stance. Second, the molded insert spreads the force on the foot over a greater surface area, limiting the pressure on more sensitive areas (Fig. 2). Because of the increased thickness of the insert, patients require extra-depth shoes. In the case of a severely dysvascular amputee who may be at increased risk of breakdown, a long steel

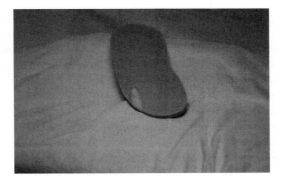

Fig. 2. Total contact insert with fourth digit toe filler.

spring shank, a metatarsal pad, or a rocker-bottom shoe may be more appropriate. The mechanics of these prosthetic components are discussed later.

Ray amputation

Ray amputations are indicated when the necrotizing or infective process requires resection of the digit and most if not all of the respective metatarsal. The loss of a ray leads to similar alterations in weight bearing and the formation of a narrower foot. Because of the transfer of weight-bearing activity to the remaining metatarsal heads, ulceration of adjacent metatarsal heads is a major long-term complication in ray resections [14]. Loss of the first toe or fifth ray, in particular, often shifts the normal weight-bearing pattern to the adjacent metatarsals, and increased skin breakdown and excessive callusing may be seen in patients at severe risk. In these cases, a shoe insert with modifications to support the metatarsal heads (metatarsal pad) and a filler for the absent rays and toes can be made if the absent ray is one not centrally located [1]. Additionally a custom-molded, flexible plantar shoe insert can be used to provide a flexible anterior extension to compensate for a missing ray to improve the rocker motion of the foot and support and protect the foot during simulated metatarsophalangeal hyperextension [15]. In a review, Maciejewski et al [13] found that patients with a severe deformity or prior history of toe or ray amputation may have significant protective effect in the prevention of further ulceration or skin breakdown on both limbs through the use of therapeutic footwear including silicone and Plastazote inserts (Zotefoams, Walton, Kentucky). The orthotic insert helps to protect the sensitive foot by providing relief for metatarsal head pressure, supports the arch to prevent foot collapse, and assists in normalizing the ground reaction pattern during terminal stance and preswing [16]. These options are sometimes expensive, however, and may be best reserved for patients at highest risk.

Transmetatarsal amputations

There are approximately 10,000 transmetatarsal amputations (TMA) per-formed in the United States each year [17]. Most authors believe that when vascular and surgical criteria can be met, a TMA is preferred over a transtibial am-putation because it preserves the ankle function, provides a distal weight-bearing surface, and creates a more energy-efficient gait [18]. A TMA also typically is preferred to a transtibial amputation because proximal levels of amputation re-quire greater energy expenditure in patients with limited cardiac function [19]. Additionally, patients who have a TMA also are more likely to ambulate inde-pendently than patients with a transtibial amputation [20].

It has been estimated that more than a quarter of patients who have undergone a TMA amputation may develop skin breakdown, with nearly a third requiring a higher level of amputation [2,18,21]. Because of the muscle imbalance created by severed dorsiflexors and the intact plantar flexors and the change in the weight-loading surface, patients who have undergone a TMA often are at increased risk of recurrent ulceration. The residual foot has a tendency to drift into equinovarus deformity as the amputation becomes more proximal, creating recurrent ulcers that are difficult to treat [8]. As mentioned earlier, as the foot becomes shorter, the ground contact and the functional lever arm of the foot decrease, which causes increased stress on the residual limb and decreased ambulation efficiency.

The biomechanical goal of prosthetic management in the TMA is to create anterior support in the area of the lost metatarsals and a fulcrum on which the foot-ankle complex pivots over the region of lost metatarsal heads in late stance phase [22]. The length and degree of flexibility of the forefoot affect the anterior lever arm and consequently foot and ankle motion. Creating too stiff an anterior lever arm may create too much pressure, however, on the amputated distal end within the socket or shoe [17].

One option available for the TMA patient, in particular limited ambulators, is a simple toe filler with a modified shoe. In this case, an extended spring steel shank or band of rigid steel is placed within the sole of the shoe, extending from the calcaneus to the metatarsal heads. As mentioned previously, the challenge for the prosthetist is to balance the appropriate degree of forefoot flexibility with the patient's needs. For a more natural-appearing and energy-efficient gate, the relative plantar rigidity should give way to at least 15° of forefoot flexibility distal to the metatarsal heads [22]. Too stiff a steel shank creates too much pressure on the metatarsal heads and causes breakdown of the forefoot.

Another option for the TMA patient, and similar to the first ray resection, is a custom-molded plantar shoe insert that incorporates a graphite or carbon fiber plate attached to the bottom of the insert. In this case, a total contact insert is fabricated over a positive cast mold from the patient's foot. Similar to the insert used in a ray resection, a medial arch support is used to prevent collapse of the longitudinal arch and prevent the foot from moving forward in the shoe, de-creasing shear (Figs. 3–5). The total contact insert maximizes the available weight-bearing surface and decreases the plantar pressures (Fig. 6) [8]. The use

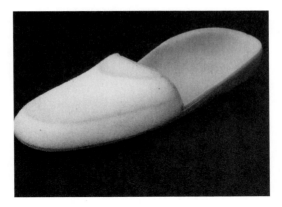

Fig. 3. Total contact transmetatarsal plastazote insert.

of a total contact insert has been shown to decrease peak plantar pressures in diabetic patients not only on the forefoot of the amputated limb, but also on the contralateral limb [23]. As mentioned previously, reduction of peak pressures on the contralateral limb is an important consideration to protect the extremity and reduce the high incidence of bilateral amputation after lower extremity amputation [24].

The newer, fabricated inserts with carbon fiber and graphite shanks also may be advantageous because they allow function similar to the spring-steel shank without requiring drastic shoe modification. Instead, they can be placed in different shoes instead of limited to a single modified shoe, while producing an improved gait pattern. Tang et al [22] found that use of a carbon-fiber plate, with toe filler and total contact insert, significantly improved gait patterns and allowed a more symmetric and cosmetic gait.

For a patient with a high risk of ulceration or chronic foot pain, a rocker-bottom shoe may provide good option for treatment of a TMA [17]. A rocker

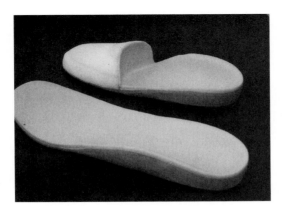

Fig. 4. Total contact transmetatarsal plastazote insert with medial arch and matching insert.

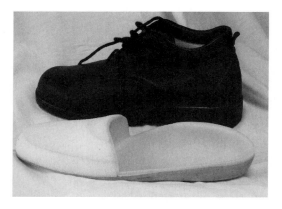

Fig. 5. Total contact transmetatarsal plastazote insert with medial arch and Apex Ambulator shoe (Aetrex Worldwide, Teaneck, New Jersey).

bottom, which is a plantar buildup that creates a curved roll, can be placed on any shoe to reduce undesirable ground reaction forces to the distal-plantar aspect of the foot and provide increased protection [8]. By placing the rocker just proximal to the distal end of the residual limb, the shoe can assist rollover and advance stance phase with a simulated toe-off making the gait more efficient. The rocker bottom helps to reduce the ground reaction force and distribute the pressure over a greater area. A high-top shoe can be incorporated in the prescription to provide additional security and used with a heel lift in more proximal TMAs that have developed an equinus deformity by better holding the foot in place and limiting the stress on the distal edge [8]. Because the rocker bottom shoe is shorter, however, it may decrease the base of support and make some patients who have more gait difficulties feel less stable and less likely to wear the shoe [25].

The ankle-foot orthosis (AFO) is another option for patients who have undergone a TMA, in particular for patients who have dynamic equinus deformity or

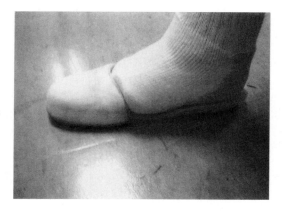

Fig. 6. TMA fit to total contact insert.

a short residual foot [8]. The AFO can be made from a plastic, copolymer shell or from a traditional double upright metal AFO with bars that are attached to a custom shoe. The plastic AFO supports the plantar aspect of the foot and extends up the back of the leg to the belly of the gastrocnemius where a circumferential strap supports the limb. The plastic AFO can be incorporated with an anterior or posterior trim line for variable ankle stability and rigidity, depending on the patient's needs. This increased rigidity and subsequent ankle restriction may be difficult, however, for some patients to tolerate. Mueller and Strube [25] found that more than 50% of the patients enrolled in a trial of various types of foot-wear for forefoot amputations refused to wear the AFO because of complaints of limited ankle motion. Of patients who tolerated the AFO, most had short residual limbs.

Because the AFO can be fitted with a total contact insert or toe filler and extended beyond the metatarsals, it provides a longer lever and a controlled fulcrum for pivoting over the lost metatarsal heads [16]. This combination can be especially valuable for a patient with a short residual limb because it can secure the heel in the shoe and limit pistoning, while creating a more efficient gait. It also is particularly useful for patients with equinovarus deformity, where the extra support of the AFO can keep the residual limb at 90° during the swing phase of gait, allowing it to contact the ground with the hind foot and limit shearing of the distal aspect of the limb [8].

Another option available for the TMA and partial foot patient is the pros-thetic boot, which has laced or Velcro ankle cuff closures that provide better attachment of the prosthesis and reduce distal motion [16]. These can be made from a wide variety of materials, ranging from plastic to leather to fabric, but they all have an anterior or medial tongue with a closure device to obtain firm attach-ment above the ankle [26]. One common option is a Chicago boot that combines a University of California Biomechanics Laboratory type (UCBL) heel cup with a toe filler attached to the prosthesis. The UCBL orthosis, which was created to treat calcaneal eversion and subtalar motion, provides better control for the foot and may help reduce shear with the bony contour of the malleolus [27].

Another device commonly used as a TMA prosthesis is the cosmetic slipper design that can be used as a cosmetic restoration and more recently as a func-tional prosthesis. In the functional prosthesis, several types are available that combine silicone sockets, polyester resins, or lamination to provide adequate support [28,29]. In one type, the Lange silicone partial foot, a silicone slipper is made from a negative impression of the residual limb and attached to a laminated silicone socket that has a zipper closure that allows easier donning and doffing [29]. The silicone slipper, or shell, sometimes is combined with an elastomer foam to create an elastic, resistive foam that allows for a smoother terminal stance. These prostheses are often ideal for swimming or water sports because the silicone is durable in the water, and the silicone allows for a flexible whip action that is useful with fins [16].

The other silicone slipper used for TMA and other partial foot amputations is a cosmetic restoration. This slipper may be appropriate for patients who place a premium on cosmesis. This prosthesis often is produced in custom manufacturing centers and can be ordered with hair, freckles, and a variety of skin tones [16]. Without additional material incorporated into the prosthesis, it provides little support. It provides little mechanical or ambulation advantage except perhaps to prolong shoe life [16].

Lisfranc's amputations

The goal of prosthetic management in a Lisfranc's amputation is similar to that of a TMA. Because the residual limb is shorter, however, certain considerations should be made to accommodate the shorter residual lever arm and for the increased risk of equinovarus deformities resulting from the unopposed force of the plantar flexors. Typically, similar options as used in a TMA prosthesis are modified to decrease the force on the residual limb during the terminal phase of gate. The prosthesis can be made with a longer toe plate to increase resistance at toe-off. Alternatively, more height can be added to the proximal portion of the prosthesis to distribute the increased force on the residual limb over a greater surface area of the plantar surface. Additionally a rocker-bottom shoe with the rocker positioned more proximally compared with a TMA can be used to provide more gait control and decrease the ground reaction forces on the distal aspect of the residual limb [30,31].

Chopart's amputation

The major advantages of a Chopart's amputation are that it offers a functional residuum with equal limb length compared with higher level amputees, and it retains ankle motion [32]. Chopart's amputation is typically a good choice for limited ambulators and patients who require stability for functional transfers. Because it has a shortened and inadequate foot lever that limits push-off and stability, however, it is typically not as effective for more active amputees [30].

Several options are available for the Chopart's amputee, but most must incorporate some additional support at or above the ankle. One such option is a full-length shoe with a prosthetic filler attached to an upright AFO. By going proximal to the malleoli, the amputee gets additional mediolateral stability. The full-length shoe extends quite far beyond the residual limb, however, and can cause increased shearing stress and ground reaction forces to the distal plantar surface, which can lead to skin breakdown [30].

A polypropylene posterior-leaf spring AFO with a custom-molded insert and molded forefoot filler is an alternative prosthetic design, which can be used for more protection and decreased stress on the residual limb. The posterior-leaf spring AFO is typically set at 90° to allow for plantar flexion after heel-strike and provide assistance with dorsiflexion of the residual foot and shoe at swing phase. The AFO has a calf strap for suspension and can be fit with an additional supramalleolar strap to prevent slippage of the residual shoe during swing phase

[30]. By using a custom polyethylene contoured to the weight-bearing surface, the prosthesis can decrease the shearing stress on the residual limb.

For Chopart's amputees who are more active, a Lange partial foot prosthesis can be used by extending the proximal portion of the prosthesis above the malleoli [30]. As with the TMA prosthesis, the silicone slipper can be combined with an elastomer foam to allow for a smoother terminal stance for the shortened residual limb. With the increased stability, the Chopart amputee is able to walk longer distances.

Syme's amputation

The major advantages of Syme's amputation over other lower extremity amputations are the ability to bear weight directly on the residual limb and the efficiency in gait compared with transtibial amputations or TMAs [32,33]. Additionally, the amputee usually can stand freely and ambulate short distances on the residual limb without the need for a prosthesis (Fig. 7) [1].

When the results are favorable, Syme's amputation is the most functional level of amputation in the lower extremity, but when the results are poor, the extremity usually must be amputated more proximally to provide the patient with adequate function or to treat the underlying vascular disease [33,34]. Two of the largest complications with this procedure are fat pad migration and poor cosmesis, but they usually can be avoided through good surgical technique [32–34]. Cosmetic complications involve wound healing and prosthetic construction.

To ensure sufficient healing of the amputation, there must be an adequate blood supply. Because of the peripheral vascular compromise commonly found in

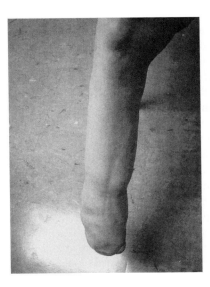

Fig. 7. Healed residual limb in a patient with a Syme's amputation.

diabetics, Syme's amputation had fallen out of favor until more recently [32]. Through judicious use of modern technology, such as Doppler ultrasound measurements of blood flow, radioactive xenon clearance tests, and transcutaneous oxygenation measurements, there has been an increase in the success rates of Syme's amputations, and it has seen a resurgence in popularity [32,33].

A patient with Syme's amputation has a decrease in the speed of ambulation by about 32% and an energy expenditure increase by about 13% compared with their able-bodied counterparts [35]. Similarly, it has been found that although transmetatarsal amputees ambulate faster than ankle disarticulation patients, individuals with ankle disarticulation amputations expend less energy during gait [36]. Pinzur et al [37] studied the gait dynamics between transmetatarsal and ankle disarticulation amputees and found that the two groups had entirely different ground reaction forces. They found that the shortened length of the residual foot in transmetatarsal amputees served as a smaller lever arm at push-off than did the full-size prosthetic foot in the ankle disarticulation amputee. Based on these results, they suggest that the midfoot amputation be used in older, more sedentary individuals, whereas an ankle disarticulation should be used in younger, more active individuals.

The design of the prosthesis for Syme's amputation is challenging in that it not only must be functional, but also cosmetically attractive. As mentioned previously, the poor cosmetic appearance of the residual limb and the subsequent prosthesis is a limiting factor behind this amputation. The poor cosmesis of the prosthesis is due in part to the fact that it must accommodate for the bulge of the residual limb, which is covered with heavy plantar skin and can be large and bulky [33]. A variation in the traditional Syme's amputation surgery consists of transecting the tibia and fibula 1.3 cm proximal to the ankle joint, leading to excision of the medial and lateral malleoli [2]. This variation leads to better cosmesis by creating a residual limb that is more uniform in diameter from proximal to distal, minimizing the formation of a distal bulbous stump and leading to a more cosmetic-appearing prosthesis [32]. In addition to conforming to the distal stump and its cosmetic characteristics, the prosthesis also must be designed to minimize contact with pressure-sensitive areas (tibial crest, lateral tibial flair, fibular head, and both malleoli), while promoting weight bearing in the tolerant regions (patella tendon, medial tibial flair, and tibialis anterior) [32].

Postoperatively the patient may be fitted with either a true prosthesis or a walking cast. The walking cast is used when one anticipates a potential for a large loss of volume, such as in peripheral edema or obesity [32]. The cast should be applied immediately after the sutures are removed, usually about 3 weeks postoperatively [32]. Four different types of prostheses commonly are fabricated today for Syme's amputation: the Canadian, medial opening, sleeve suspension, and flexible wall design [32].

The Canadian design consists of a removable posterior panel to ease donning and doffing and is one of the most cosmetic of the available choices. This design is cosmetic because it does not have any additional buildup or hardware around the ankle. The tradeoff with this design is that prosthesis breakage and failure are higher because the posterior cutout at the ankle weakens the ankle, which undergoes the most tension during ambulation [32].

The medial opening prosthesis (Fig. 8) is also known as the Veterans Administration Prosthetic Center prosthesis [32]. Compared with the posterior design, the medial opening design also is cosmetic, but it additionally provides more stability at the ankle, and it is more durable and is the usual choice for patients with Syme's amputation [30]. Patients who need a stronger prosthesis, such as obese patients or patients who perform heavy manual labor, benefit from a sleeve suspension–type prosthesis. This type of prosthesis also commonly is referred to as a "stovepipe" prosthesis and consists of a flexible inner sleeve that slides into the prosthetic shell, resembling an exoskeletal transtibial prosthesis. Because there are no windows cut into the prosthesis, it is stronger than the Canadian and medial opening [1], but the added bulk makes it less cosmetic [32].

The final type of prosthesis is the expandable wall prosthesis. This prosthesis consists of an inner socket wall that expands to accommodate the entry of the residual limb. When the limb is inside, the socket contracts to provide total contact to the residual limb. The expandable wall makes this prosthesis more bulky than the Canadian and medial opening styles, but the ease of donning and doffing makes it the choice for individuals with upper extremity or cognitive impairments [32]. Despite the fact that newer technologies, such as thermoplastics and silicone elastomers, have made this prosthesis lighter and more

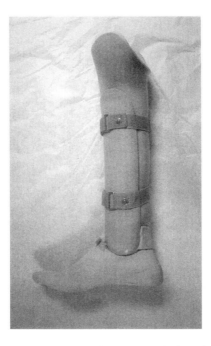

Fig. 8. Medial opening molded plastic Symes prosthesis with a SACH foot.

durable, it is still more challenging to fabricate and is more difficult to adjust than the other types previously mentioned [1,32].

The Syme's prosthesis uses the same type of prosthetic foot options as used in the traditional transtibial prosthesis, such as the stationary ankle flexible endoskeletal (SAFE) foot and solid ankle cushion heel (SACH) foot. These feet must be constructed with a lower profile to accommodate for the longer residual limb [33]. Although the SACH foot is the most traditional foot used in the Syme's prosthesis, other types, such as the SAFE foot and energy-storing models, also are used routinely depending on the patient's strength, mobility, and daily activities [32]. The aforementioned low profile results in locking of the ankle, leading to a higher degree of work of the quadriceps muscles during the loading response of gait [32]. The demand on the quadriceps muscle can be lessened by adjusting the ankle to a few degrees of plantar flexion [32]. The typical foot is set in 5° of dorsiflexion to mimic normal gait patterns, but as mentioned earlier, a slight plantarward adjustment may be necessary in individuals with quadriceps weakness, to prevent knee buckling [32]. This additional plantar flexion puts the ground reaction force in front of the knee to make the knee more stable.

The positioning of the socket also is designed to mimic normal gait patterns. Because the patient with Syme's amputation still retains most of the tibia and fibula, the socket is designed at an "angle of adduction" equivalent to the anatomic adduction of the tibia [32]. The prosthesis should fit such that there is a 12-mm varus moment at the knee to simulate normal gait mechanics [32]. This varus moment is established through the functional alignment of the socket adduction angle, foot eversion angle, and linear displacement [32]. Because any variation from this alignment would result in an inefficient and noncosmetic gait pattern, it takes an experienced prosthetist to recognize and correct malalignments.

As mentioned earlier, Syme's amputation has seen a resurgence thanks to the help of improved medical and surgical techniques, along with advancements in prosthetic technology. Prosthetic fitting of the patient with Syme's amputation can be challenging and requires an experienced prosthetist to determine which style would be most beneficial to the patient. When properly fitted, however, these patients should be able to ambulate efficiently and perform their activities of daily living without much difficulty.

Summary

Partial foot amputations provide challenges and advantages to the physician confronting a patient with a limb loss. Because the partial foot amputee often can bear weight and has a more energy-efficient gait, there are many opportunities available to the prosthetic team. As with any prosthetic prescription for a patient with limb loss, the goals of the rehabilitation team are to maintain function, prevent further deformity, and restore function as much as possible. Numerous options are available for each level of pedal amputee, but designing and fitting a prosthetic socket that is comfortable and meets the needs of the individual is the key to the prescription. The prescribing physician should keep in mind the alteration in amputee gait, its resultant change in weight-bearing surface, and, most importantly, the needs and expectations of the amputee to ensure that the prosthesis is functional and well used.

References

[1] Leonard JA, Meier J, Meier RH. Upper and lower extremity prosthetics. In: DeLisa JA, Gans BM, editors. Rehabilitation medicine: principles and practice. Philadelphia: Lippincott-Raven; 1998. p. 669–96.

[2] Mueller MJ, Salsich GB, Bastian AJ. Differences in the gait characteristics of people with diabetes and transmetatarsal amputation compared with age-matched contols. Gait Posture 1998; 70:200–6.

[3] Saunders JB, Inman VT, Eberhart HD. The major determinants in normal and pathologic gait. J Bone Joint Surg 1953;35A:543–58.

[4] Wright DG, Desai M, Henderson WH. Action of the subtalar and ankle-joint complex during the stance phase of walking. J Bone Joint Surg 1964;46A:361–82.

[5] Nole R, Garbalosa JC. Foot and ankle prosthetics. In: Lusardi M, editor. Orthotics and prosthetics in rehabilitation. Boston: Butterworth-Heinemann; 2000. p. 129–58.

[6] Pinzur M, Gold J, Schwartz D, et al. Energy demands for walking in dysvascular amputees as related to the level of amputation. Orthopaedics 1992;15:1033–7.

[7] Hirsch G, McBride ME, Murray DD, et al. Chopart prosthesis and semirigid foot orthosis in traumatic forefoot amputation: comparative gait analysis. Am J Phys Med Rehabil 1996; 75:283–91.

[8] Catanzarti AR, Medicino RW, Haverstock B. Considerations for protection of the residual foot following transmetatarsal amputation. Wounds 1999;11:13–20.

[9] Burnfield JM, Boyd LA, Rao S, et al. The effect of partial foot amputation on sound limb loading force during barefoot walking. Gait Posture 1998;7:178–9.

[10] Leonard JA. Lower limb prosthetic sockets. Phys Med Rehabil State Art Rev 1994;8:129–45.

[11] Funk C, Young G. Subtotal pedal amputations: biomechanical and intraoperative considerations. J Am Podiatr Med Assoc 2001;91:6–12.

[12] Lavery LA, Lavery DC, Quebedeaux-Farnham TL. Increased foot pressures after great toe amputation in diabetes. Diabetes Care 1995;19:1460–2.

[13] Maciejewski ML, Reiber GE, Smith DG, et al. Effectiveness of diabetic therapeutic footwear in preventing reulceration. Diabetes Care 2004;27:1774–82.

[14] Gianfortune P, Pulla RJ, Sage R. Ray resections in the insensitive or dysvascular foot: a critical review. J Foot Surg 1985;24:103–7.

[15] Young RD. Special Chopart prosthesis with custom molded foot. Orthot Prosthet 1984;38: 79–85.

[16] Ayyappa E. Postsurgical management of partial foot and Syme's amputation. In: Lusardi M, editor. Orthotics and prosthetics in rehabilitation. Boston: Butterworth-Heinemann; 2000. p. 379–93.

[17] National Center for Health Statistics. National hospital discharge survey, 1991. Hyattsville (MD): National Center for Health Statistics; 1993.

[18] Mueller MJ, Allen BT, Sinacore DR. Incidence of skin break-down and higher amputation after transmetatarsal amputation: Implications for rehabilitation. Arch Phys Med Rehabil 1995;76: 50–4.

[19] Waters RL, Perry J, Antonelli D, et al. Energy cost of walking amputees: influence of level of amputation. J Bone Joint Surg 1976;58(A):42–7.

[20] Miller N, Allen BT, Sinacore DR. Transmetatarsal amputation: the role of adjunctive re-vasularization. J Vasc Surg 1991;13:705–11.
[21] Durham JR, McCoy DM, Sawchuk AP, et al. Open transmetatarsal amputation in the treatment of severe foot infections. Am J Surg 1989;158:127–30.
[22] Tang SF, Chen CPC, Chen MHL, et al. Transmetatasal amputation prosthesis with carbon-fiberplate: enhanced gait function. Am J Phys Med Rehabil 2004;83:124–30.
[23] Mueller MJ, Strube MJ, Allen BT. Therapeutic footwear can reduce plantar pressures in pa-tients with diabetes and tranmetarsal amputation. Diabetes Care 1997;20:637–41.
[24] Pecoraro RE, Reiber GE, Burgess EM. Pathways to diabetic limb amputation: basis for pre-vention. Diabetes Care 1990;13:513–21.
[25] Mueller MJ, Strube MJ. Therapeutic footwear: enhanced function in people with diabetes and transmetatarsal amputation. Arch Phys Med Rehabil 1997;78:952–6.
[26] Collins JN. Partial foot prosthesis for the transmetatarsal level. Clin Prosthet Orthot 1987–1998; 12:19–23.
[27] Imler CD. Imler partial foot prosthesis: IPFP—the Chicago boot. Orthot Prosthet 1985;39: 53–6.
[28] Stills M. Partial foot prosthesis/orthosis. Clin Prosthet Orthot 1987–1988;2:14–8.
[29] Lange RL. The Lange silicone partial foot prosthesis. J Prosthet Orthot 1992;4:56.
[30] Philbin TM, Leyes M, Sferra JJ, et al. Orthotic and prosthetic devices in partial foot amputa-tions. Foot Ankle Clin 2001;6:215–28.
[31] Parziale JR, Hahn KA. Function considerations in partial foot amputations. Orthop Rev 1988; 17:262–6.
[32] Lusardi MM, Nielsen CC. Foot and ankle prosthetics. In: Lusardi M, editor. Orthotics and prosthetics in rehabilitation. Boston: Butterworth-Heinemann; 2000. p. 386–93.
[33] Richardson EG. Amputations about the feet. In: Canale ST, editor. Campbell's operative orthopaedics. 10th edition. Philadelphia: Mosby; 2003. p. 556–71.
[34] Pinzur MS, Pinzur RM, Stuck R, et al. Syme ankle disarticulation in patients with diabetes. J Bone Joint Surg Am 2003;85:1667–72.
[35] Leonard EI. Lower limb prostheses. In: Braddom RL, editor. Physical medicine and reha-bilitation. Philadelphia: WB Saunders; 2000. p. 279–310.
[36] Pinzur M, Gold J, Schwartz D, et al. Energy demands for walking in dysvascular amputees as related to the level of amputation. Orthopaedics 1992;15:1033–7.
[37] Pinzur M, Wolf B, Havey R. Walking pattern of midfoot and ankle disarticulation ampu-tees. Foot Ankle Int 1997;18:635–8.

ELSEVIER
SAUNDERS

Clin Podiatr Med Surg
22 (2005) 503–508

CLINICS IN
PODIATRIC
MEDICINE AND
SURGERY

Index

Note: Page numbers of article titles are in **boldface** type.

Changing Your Address?

Make sure your subscription changes too! When you notify us of your new address, you can help make our job easier by including an exact copy of your Clinics label number with your old address (see illustration below.) This number identifies you to our computer system and will speed the processing of your address change. Please be sure this label number accompanies your old address and your corrected address—you can send an old Clinics label with your number on it or just copy it exactly and send it to the address listed below.

We appreciate your help in our attempt to give you continuous coverage. Thank you.

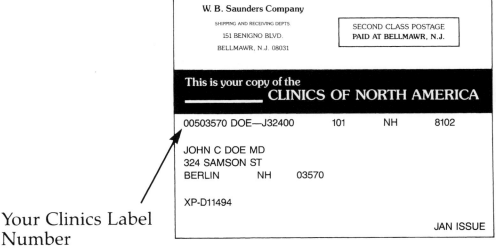

Your Clinics Label Number

Copy it exactly or send your label
along with your address to:
W.B. Saunders Company, Customer Service
Orlando, FL 32887-4800
Call Toll Free 1-800-654-2452

Please allow four to six weeks for delivery of new subscriptions and for processing address changes.

Order your subscription today. Simply complete and detach this card and drop it in the mail to receive the best clinical information in your field.

Please Print:

Name _____

Address _____

City_____ State _____ ZIP _____

Method of Payment

❏ Check (payable to **Elsevier**; add the applicable sales tax for your area)

❏ VISA   ❏ MasterCard   ❏ AmEx   ❏ Bill me

Card number _____ Exp. date _____

Signature _____

Staple this to your purchase order to expedite delivery

Adolescent Medicine Clinics
- ❏ Individual $95
- ❏ Institutions $133
- ❏ *In-training $48

Anesthesiology
- ❏ Individual $175
- ❏ Institutions $270
- ❏ *In-training $88

Cardiology
- ❏ Individual $170
- ❏ Institutions $266
- ❏ *In-training $85

Chest Medicine
- ❏ Individual $185
- ❏ Institutions $285

Child and Adolescent Psychiatry
- ❏ Individual $175
- ❏ Institutions $265
- ❏ *In-training $88

Critical Care
- ❏ Individual $165
- ❏ Institutions $266
- ❏ *In-training $83

Dental
- ❏ Individual $150
- ❏ Institutions $242

Emergency Medicine
- ❏ Individual $170
- ❏ Institutions $263
- ❏ *In-training $85
- ❏ Send CME info

Facial Plastic Surgery
- ❏ Individual $199
- ❏ Institutions $300

Foot and Ankle
- Individual $160
- Institutions $232

Gastroenterology
- ❏ Individual $190
- ❏ Institutions $276

Gastrointestinal Endoscopy
- ❏ Individual $190
- ❏ Institutions $276

Hand
- ❏ Individual $205
- ❏ Institutions $319

Heart Failure (NEW in 2005!)
- ❏ Individual $99
- ❏ Institutions $149
- ❏ *In-training $49

Hematology/ Oncology
- ❏ Individual $210
- ❏ Institutions $315

Immunology & Allergy
- ❏ Individual $165
- ❏ Institutions $266

Infectious Disease
- ❏ Individual $165
- ❏ Institutions $272

Clinics in Liver Disease
- ❏ Individual $165
- ❏ Institutions $234

Medical
- ❏ Individual $140
- ❏ Institutions $244
- ❏ *In-training $70
- ❏ Send CME info

MRI
- ❏ Individual $190
- ❏ Institutions $290
- ❏ *In-training $95
- ❏ Send CME info

Neuroimaging
- ❏ Individual $190
- ❏ Institutions $290
- ❏ *In-training $95
- ❏ Send CME info

Neurologic
- ❏ Individual $175
- ❏ Institutions $275

Obstetrics & Gynecology
- ❏ Individual $175
- ❏ Institutions $288

Occupational and Environmental Medicine
- ❏ Individual $120
- ❏ Institutions $166
- ❏ *In-training $60

Ophthalmology
- ❏ Individual $190
- ❏ Institutions $325

Oral & Maxillofacial Surgery
- ❏ Individual $180
- ❏ Institutions $280
- ❏ *In-training $90

Orthopedic
- ❏ Individual $180
- ❏ Institutions $295
- ❏ *In-training $90

Otolaryngologic
- ❏ Individual $199
- ❏ Institutions $350

Pediatric
- ❏ Individual $135
- ❏ Institutions $246
- ❏ *In-training $68
- ❏ Send CME info

Perinatology
- ❏ Individual $155
- ❏ Institutions $237
- ❏ *In-training $78
- ❏ Send CME info

Plastic Surgery
- ❏ Individual $245
- ❏ Institutions $370

Podiatric Medicine & Surgery
- ❏ Individual $170
- ❏ Institutions $266

Primary Care
- ❏ Individual $135
- ❏ Institutions $223

Psychiatric
- ❏ Individual $170
- ❏ Institutions $288

Radiologic
- ❏ Individual $220
- ❏ Institutions $331
- ❏ *In-training $110
- ❏ Send CME info

Sports Medicine
- ❏ Individual $180
- ❏ Institutions $277

Surgical
- ❏ Individual $190
- ❏ Institutions $299
- ❏ *In-training $95

Thoracic Surgery (formerly Chest Surgery)
- ❏ Individual $175
- ❏ Institutions $255
- ❏ *In-training $88

Urologic
- ❏ Individual $195
- ❏ Institutions $307
- ❏ *In-training $98
- ❏ Send CME info

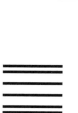